Caregiving from the Trenches

A true story about a woman's journey of
caregiving and self-discovery

Alexandra Lindquist

This book is not intended as a substitute for the medical advice of physicians. The reader should regularly consult a physician in matters relating to his/her health and particularly with respect to any symptoms that may require diagnosis or medical attention.

No part of this publication may be reproduced, stored in a retrieval system, or transmitted in any form or by any means, electronic, mechanical, photocopying, recording, or otherwise, without expressed written permission of the author, Alexandra Lindquist.

TABLE OF CONTENTS

ACKNOWLEDGMENTS

Thank you to my daughter, for proofreading and support
throughout the writing and publishing process.
Thank you to my husband, for being an inspiration and for
your unwavering support. For teaching me how to be
stronger and more independent, and for showing me how
to cope with life with grace and humor.

1 PREFACE

No one knows what life will bring. There are times bad things happen. Being able to cope with life when your loved ones get sick is hard. It's difficult so see them sick and you are virtually helpless. You cannot cure them but you can make them feel a little better when you look after them, even if it's for a short period of time.

Making appointments for them, relieving them from some of the workload, or just sitting with them, can make them feel at ease and cope with their problems and how they are feeling. Let them express their feelings and what they are going through in terms of the pain or frustration they feel. It's difficult to hear but patience and understanding is required. Some days will be better than others and as a caregiver you need to listen and hear what they say and not blame them or get angry.

The gamut of emotions a caregiver goes through is horrendous. One does not realize how hard it is until you go through it and it seems it goes on forever but it does end sometime. The stress a caregiver goes through may cause chronic illnesses and when that happens you need to talk to your doctor. You too will need medication and supplements during your caregiving days if you don't practice self-care. They have done studies that prove chronic illnesses occur when you are under a lot of stress and pressure over an extended period of time, and sometimes it just happens.

As a caregiver you will feel unappreciated and your loved ones will take you for granted. It isn't their fault, they don't see what it's doing to you, and it's understandable from their point, after all they are the ones that are sick. Get good at hiding your feelings when you are dealing with your loved one. It isn't fair on them to make them feel guilty but do find someone you can talk to it can make all the difference. There are hot lines for caregivers, that I didn't use, online resources, I didn't use, or talking to your family doctor about what you're going through, which I didn't. it was my mistake and I regret it because I needed help and didn't get it. I don't think my bouts of depression would not have been as difficult or as long as they were if I had only sought out help for myself. I thought it was a weakness to admit that it was too much of a burden. Looking back, I realize it wasn't a weakness but a normal reaction when placed under that much stress. Use the resources available, they could save your life and your sanity.

You will have good days and bad days, just don't let your loved one know, it's hard enough on them dealing with their illness and how they feel. As each day passes, it will get easier for you especially if you see them getting a little better every day, as was the case with my husband, we didn't notice how well he was doing until an entire year had gone by. He could do so much more by the end of one year. With my father, he would not do anything to get better and over the years he required more assistance as time went on. My husband wanted his independence back and my father wanted nothing more than for me to do everything for him.

Each individual is different, only you will be able to tell what you can do to help. Some may require a little push and others may not want to help themselves at all. You will be the judge for what you need to do to help them deal with it. Don't make it harder on them than it already is. Trust me on this, they feel bad about what they are feeling and doing to you, they will never admit it, but some of the anger you will experience coming from your loved one is the guilt they feel for getting sick.

Try to keep the everyday things away from them like paying bills, household duties, shopping, or even working. It will take much longer for them to get better if they too are stressed all of the time.

Research the illness so you know what is happening with them. There are so many online resources, doctors, nurses, hospitals, and even pharmacies. All you have to do is look and you will find the information you need to help your loved one cope. There isn't much available that I could find on what the caregiver goes through but it is out there if you're persistent enough. It's important for you as a caregiver to look after yourself and learn coping mechanisms that work for you. You cannot be a good caregiver if you aren't looking after yourself. Be kind to yourself, after all you're only human too.

If you are looking after both parents, I found that the other one becomes jealous of the time you give to the one that is actually sick. If and when this happens, you will need to learn to manage your time equally between them, it is doable, but very difficult to deal with. On one hand you want to give your undivided attention to the person that is actually sick and then the other one pretends to need you but you still have to deal with the situation.

Over the years I found I changed, I became stronger and more independent. You don't see the changes from day to day but after several years you realize you are not the same person you were when it all started. I gained more patience and understanding. I don't fly off the handle as much as I used to and use breathing exercises to relieve the stress and pressure when someone pushes my buttons. When my husband pushed me to my limits he soon learned if I used the phrase 'yes dear', he would back off and walk away. I could regain my strength and carry on without getting angry at him. I know it was hard for him at the start and he required a lot of assistance doing anything but I wanted him to get his independence back in hopes of him feeling better about himself.

When a person doesn't feel good about themselves, they go out of their way to make the other person angry or put them down. Don't fall into their trap. Walk away and realize they didn't mean what they said and come back with a smile on your face. If they know it doesn't affect you, they will stop doing it after a while.

With my parents, they didn't see the tell-tale signs and didn't really care if I was angry, so they kept on doing it. I was raised to never show your feelings if I was angry at them. They always thought they were perfect and did no wrong. Still today I cannot tell my mother that she is doing something that annoys me or has gone too far. She takes the offensive immediately and at that point she doesn't listen, instead she attacks.

I've made sure my daughter can talk to me like she would talk to anyone that annoys her. I always taught her to stand up for herself and speak out if something or someone is bothering her. It is hard not to be able to tell a parent that they are hurting you or making you unhappy. Keeping it inside only causes problems in the long run and you begin to resent them for it. As a caregiver you should still be able to tell the person you are looking after that what they are doing is making you miserable and that they should stop, but if you can't their behavior never changes.

I took it out on my husband when I was frustrated with my parents but it wasn't fair to him because he was not part of the problem. I had to find an outlet for my anger other than my husband, he too was sick and didn't need the stress of seeing me angry about the situation with my parents. He didn't like what they were doing to me and neither of us could fix it, we just had to live with it and get past it.

I learned a technique to relieve my stress and it was just so easy I couldn't believe it, I made sure that when I was out, I would tell complete strangers to have a great day, not just a good day, it made me feel better being kind to someone you don't know because you don't know what they're life is like. Maybe their life was even more stressful than mine but I always got a great response from them. Kindness goes along way and somehow their day is better and so is yours. It doesn't cost anything to give a kind word or smile to a stranger and life will look brighter for everyone. When I'm standing in line and it's busy, if someone behind me has a few items and I have a full buggy, I let them go ahead. The response you get is amazing, they are grateful and say something nice, usually, about your kind deed. I don't' look to get anything back when I do something nice for someone it just makes me feel better doing it.

I've even had people tell me their life story while out shopping, people are for the most part good and kind if that's what you expect, if you think they're not, chances are they won't be. How you perceive the world, that's how the world will perceive you.

I talked to people when I was waiting for my husband or my father's doctor appointment. They were as grateful as I was that we could talk to someone else other than the loved ones we were both looking after. Talking about nothing in particular, I found both parties walk away smiling, making the day seem cheerier somehow.

Anger and depression are the emotions a caregiver will experience the most. It is such an unrewarding job. Your loved ones do not know how much stress you are under because of their illness. You do so much more because of it, working, looking after the person, on top of your own regular duties. At the time I was going through it, I could not see an end to it, I thought I would be doing it for the rest of my life and then one day, it was over and the storm above me cleared up.

Every year I got depressed and angry. When these emotions took over, I went out of my way to be kind to strangers, friends, and family, and I would feel better. I never let myself get too depressed because I would be of no use to anyone, including myself. These emotions are wasteful, they destroy your well-being, and deprive you of having a good day, week, or month. Negative feelings cannot and will not let you enjoy your life, even if you aren't a caregiver, it is still a waste of time and energy.

I know of a few other women who are going through the same thing as I am. One lady has small children at home and stays at her parent's house when one parent gets sick. The parents refuse to look after each other as was the case with mine. I don't understand this at all, as long as they are both living the child should not have the burden of looking after his/her parents. It is unfair to the child. I never put that burden on mine and I never will. As long as my husband and I are alive, we will look after each other to the best of our ability. So far, the burden has been on me, but no one knows what the future will bring, and maybe he will have to tend to my needs down the road.

I've included funny stories at the back of the book. The stories occurred during this period and there were a lot of humorous events. Not all of the days were bad and as time went on, there were fewer and fewer bad days. It's all about the way you look at life.

I've also included some websites that may be of some use to you, check them out when you need help or you want more information. There are also sample forms at the back you will need for the hospital. I've included the websites for these forms and you can download and print them out.

Emotions of the Year – Working Pages

Your loved one has just had a life changing event, or been given a frightening diagnosis. Do you feel angry? Scared? Frustrated? Like crying? Helpless? If you answered "yes" to any or all of the above, you're not the only one. Being a caregiver is one of the hardest jobs a person can do. Here are some suggestions for handling the emotions above.

Do you feel angry?

Stop, walk away for a few moments, and think of something funny that happened, and try to laugh about that situation. It will make you less angry for a while. Grab a sheet of paper and write down why you're angry.

Start with this: I am angry because:

Do you feel scared?

Everyone gets scared that they will lose their loved ones, I know I did. Often, we can ignore it, but when that life-changing event happens, or that frightening diagnosis is received, suddenly we are looking mortality in the eye. Don't dwell on the loss, instead think of all the great times, the fun times, and the new things that you will do with that person. Enjoy being with them now.

I am scared because:

Do you feel frustrated?

I felt like pulling my hair out. My loved ones wouldn't listen, or hear me, or care about what I was saying. I get it, were the ones going through it, not me, but I was affected because I love them and because it would fall to me to take care of them. Go to another room, take a walk (if possible), grab a book and read for a while. Do something to take your mind off it.

I feel frustrated because:

Do you feel like crying?

Never ever let them see you cry. They already feel bad. Lock yourself in the bathroom until the moment passes and/or you have a good cry. Just make sure you wait long enough that you won't cry when you're around them. Trust me, they feel bad about the situation too.

I feel like crying because:

Do you feel helpless?

You want to do everything for them, but you shouldn't. They also feel helpless and often they feel guilty for needing your help. They aren't allowed to do things that they used to and they feel useless. Allow them to do the things that are within their abilities. Don't try to make them do things they are uncomfortable doing or fearful of. If you can, as the caregiver, take some time and do something for yourself. Self-care is important. Even if it's fifteen minutes, you'll feel better. Find the time, it's crucial for you to look after yourself. After all, if you get run down, or ill, who will take care of your loved one?

I feel helpless because:

_____

2 TIME MANAGEMENT

Making time for yourself is the hardest thing to do. Start by taking five minutes and increasing it over a period of time. When you start doing it you will find it isn't as hard as you think. Your mind needs the rest. Too much stress about your loved one will make you sick too. I know, that's what happened to me.

Grab your favorite beverage and stare out a window for five minutes and let your mind go blank. At first, it's hard to find five minutes but as each day goes by you will be able to gain a few more minutes and before you know it an hour has passed by.

There are simple tricks that let you gain quiet time for yourself. Get a white board if you can, a daily planner, or even a scribbler. Keep track of the days you need to take your loved one to the doctor, ordering pills, and when you pick up the medications. This also helps everyone in the house know what you are doing or where you are going to be at all times. Still to this day I use my white board and a daily planner. I don't have to worry about if I forgot something that day because it's written down and in plain sight.

Keep a log handy so you can jot down when your loved one isn't feeling good, time, event, and what they felt, this way you can show their doctor what was happening to them. The doctors found this information very useful. You don't have to keep a daily log and say they felt fine or were doing well, but the bad days are good to have written down, there is no way you can remember all of them before your next doctor's visit. Use a scribbler, notepad, or a pocket calendar, anything that is handy.

When you're at the pharmacy check around for a pill box, they're inexpensive and depending on the quantity of pills, you may want to get several. I had enough pill boxes for a month. Sorting pills out for a month gains you a lot of time daily. My husband was taking thirteen pills a day and it was very time consuming to take one pill out of each bottle every day. If the bottles are already open, it takes only a few minutes and you are done for the month. Also check for a pill cutter at the pharmacy if you are cutting up his or her pills. Pharmacies also offer blister packs at no additional cost to you. These blister packs contain all the pills your loved one takes and which times but it takes longer for the pharmacy to put it together so be prepared to wait, unless you order them beforehand.

If you are not happy with a certain pharmacy, find another one. Letting them get to know you and you them is important. Whenever my father was released from the hospital and I had a new prescription to fill, I would take it in immediately and the pharmacists would fill it right away. There was no waiting, which was good because my father had problems sitting in the vehicle for any length of time, he just wanted to go home. I switched pharmacies a few times until I found one that was a perfect fit for me.

When you are at the hospital, they usually ask for a list of medications, the pharmacy can give you a printout, or keep a list on a card, my daughter made a card for her Dad with all his pills and updates it when something changes, or maybe put the list on your phone.

A baby monitor helps to let you know when your loved one wakes up during the day. I didn't think of it right away but when I got one, I found I wasn't running up and down the stairs to check on my father, I only had to keep the monitor close by. I could sit outside or do whatever I wanted to until he woke up, this saved me a lot of time and energy, and wear and tear on my knees.

When cooking meals, make enough so that you can put some in the freezer. If you're really busy you can take it out and defrost it. I always make more than one day's worth and freeze some, so on the days when I get home late, it's just a matter of going to the freezer. My husband does not like eating out and gets upset if I get a pizza or any fast food, so I learned to cook a larger quantity for days when I get home late and now it's less time cooking and I have more time for myself. Shopping online for groceries, Skip the Dishes, and Chef's Plate are also possibilities for gaining time, these were not available to me when I was a caregiver.

Put together a schedule for yourself for the day, week, and even for the month. If you know what needs doing for the day when you get up, you can plan for it. Try to make doctor's appointments for the morning, they aren't too far behind in their schedule. I have yet to meet a doctor that keeps on his schedule, even if you are their first appointment. Less time waiting will gain you more time in the long run. Some appointments can't be changed. I get a letter in the mail for my husband's cardiologist every year and he only see's patients on Thursday afternoons, but I ask for the first appointment after lunch. Doctors always get behind, so earlier is better whether it's in the morning or afternoon.

Check the status of everyone's medication, that way you can order them before they run out. Twice my mother didn't inform me of my father's insulin running out and it was the worst scenario weather-wise, a blinding snow storm, when I had to drive out and pick it up. I started to keep track of his pills and insulin after that.

Learn to do things more quickly. It used to take me six hours to scrub the floors but I learned to do them under three hours. I cut the time down and freed up more time for myself or other things I could accomplish during the day. Learn to be more efficient, it really does help.

Don't put off what you need to do. You don't know what tomorrow will bring. No procrastinating. Prioritize everything that needs doing and do them in order of importance. If it isn't high on the list, don't worry about it there will be time to do it down the road or it may not matter if you ever get to it.

Plan ahead. You'll find that some things aren't

important. I used to clean out the closets twice a year. Now I do it when I have nothing else to do. Sometimes it's every other year. It isn't a priority anymore and it really doesn't matter when I get to it.

Learn to say 'no'. You'll find that your loved ones may put more demands on you because you have been doing a lot for them and will expect you to do even more. Some things they are capable of doing themselves. Get them to do it even if they don't want to. I could not convince my father to do anything for himself no matter what I did or said. He refused to go for walks because it hurt but he may have lived longer if he did. I knew it hurt but if he had started walking it would have become much easier for him every day.

Don't be afraid to ask for help. I found out from our doctor that if a person is really sick, a nurse can come out and help for the day or take their bloodwork instead of you having to drive them to a medical centre, even if you live in the country. It was hard for my father to sit in a waiting room after fasting all night, so having someone come out to the house was better for him and also for me.

Organization is the key for time. Get organized and stay organized and you will have gained all the time you need to look after yourself because that's what really important for you. You cannot help your loved one if you get sick too. Do not get to this point.

3 SELF-CARE

This is the most important thing you need to do. One of the problems that arise if you don't look after yourself is caregiver's burnout. There were a few times I experienced it. I was completely useless but I still worked through it. It was hard to do anything for my loved ones or myself. They relied on me and I just didn't want to do it. I worked through it but if I would have asked for help instead of doing everything myself, I would have gotten over the burnout much quicker or it wouldn't have happened at all. Looking after yourself is a necessity, not a luxury.

Make sure you are eating at regular times, no matter what is going on around you. Without proper sustenance your mood will change and you will become depressed. Check with your doctor if you need to take vitamin supplements, sometimes the meals don't have everything in them that your body requires or you may need a new medication to make you feel better.

Taking the time to shower or bath will make you feel much better and don't worry about your loved one, they will be fine for an hour. Let your mind go blank and enjoy the hot water, it will feel like you washed all your troubles down the drain.

Sit down with a cup of coffee and stare out into space. Your mind also needs to heal and have quiet moments too. Your brain is a muscle and it needs to rest and recharge. If you don't, you will lose concentration and focus. A scattered brain will not help anyone. Take a nap, let your mind wander, or take a walk if possible. I take my coffee first thing in the morning and sit outside during summer days and read my book, there are many ideas online to help you. Not every idea is for you but find some things that will help. Find an activity that works for you, one that you can lose yourself in. I look for quiet, alone time. It really does help. I find it easier to cope for the rest of my hectic day.

Try doing something you can focus on. Go to a book store, treat yourself to fuzzy slippers, buy something you like, it doesn't have to be expensive. Doing something for yourself will make you feel better. Put on a nice outfit, makeup, or give yourself a facial. No one else is going to pamper you, take some time for yourself and enjoy the moment. You have earned a reward, treat it as one, and don't feel guilty about it.

Make time for yourself, this will make you a happier and healthier person, if you don't, you may develop chronic stress, high blood pressure, or even diabetes. Many chronic illnesses have been proven, occur from too much stress over a long period.

Call a friend, chatting about anything else besides caregiving is a distraction from your life and will allow your mind to recharge.

Yoga and meditation are great for your mind and body too. There are many exercises online to guide you through them. I found a set of cards at the book store that showed me different positions in yoga that helped me relax. I still do it today.

Laughter is still the best medicine. Find things that make you smile or laugh. Still to this day, whenever I sit down, I break out laughing at something funny that happened or I heard and no one is home with me but it makes the world seem a bit brighter. My daughter has caught me laughing by myself many times and says, "there's Mom, again, laughing at the kitchen." There are times I laugh so hard I end up waking everyone up in the house.

I found 'YOUTUBE' to have the funniest animal videos and made a shortcut on my computer so I can watch them whenever I want and not have to do a search every time. When I'm feeling down or blue, I sit down and watch them and then I feel better. There are many sites online if you're computer savvy or find a comic book for yourself, or even a joke book. Anything you can think of that will make you laugh.

Everything that I talked about and many more that I haven't covered are available online and will definitely help you achieve these goals. Never forget a well-rested mind and body will allow you to give your loved ones all the attention they need. Look after yourself, this should become the most important thing to do for them and yourself.

4 DEATH

Make sure you have a copy of the will or living will. You cannot get a death certificate without one.

I knew what my father's last wishes were because we discussed it prior to his passing. It isn't a comfortable topic but it needed to be said so I would know what to do when it happened. The worst outcome from caring for your loved ones is death. My father passed away in 2014 and I never knew what was required for a funeral. The day after he died, the hospital called and asked where they could ship my father's body. This wasn't something I thought would happen so quickly. I knew where he wanted his resting place to be, which helped.

The next day the funeral home called to find out the details. My mother was not able to help or answer any questions. I made all the decisions on this matter. Funeral homes break it down in small increments and explain everything that's going to happen. They are very helpful and kind. It wasn't as difficult as I thought. I was never required to put together a funeral but the funeral directors knew what to do and prepared me for what happens next. My father died on a Saturday and by Tuesday the funeral took place. It all happened so fast and it was over.

The funeral directors gave me a binder with all the crucial details including where you need to send copies of the death certificate and who to inform. Doctors, lawyers, banks, pharmacies, and credit card companies need to know the person passed away as soon as possible. This I found to be very useful. One does not realize how many people need to be informed of their passing, this way, identity theft is less likely to happen and this seems to happen more often than one knows, protect yourself.

You will have to file a final tax return for them and include a death certificate. When I applied for my father's death certificate the DMV wanted my parent's marriage certificate and immigration papers. My father had destroyed the papers I needed years before, and this became a big problem. I could not produce the required documents. I went to another DMV and had no problem getting a death certificate. Don't panic if one DMV will not release what you need. Go to another one until you get the right result.

Dealing with their belongings after their passing is a subject that is hard to bring up with other family members. Everyone is different, go with your gut feelings on this matter about when you can broach the subject. This is a very uncomfortable matter, be cautious and don't take offense if the surviving spouse isn't ready to deal with it, you can always do it later, when they are ready.

Now the time came, a few months later, when I had to talk to my mother about removing the contents of his bedroom. It was a hard thing to do but it needed doing. There are places you can drop off the furniture and clothing rather than taking everything to the dump. Some churches will pick up most furniture items at no cost to you and they pass it on to people in need. There are bins in most shopping centers where you can deposit clothing and sundry items. Drop them off while on a shopping trip saving you some time.

There are so many things you need to do while being a caregiver and many more after they have passed away that no one realizes.

5 CAREGIVERS BURNOUT

If you have caregiver's burnout, you will experience symptoms such as, fatigue, irritability, drinking too much, smoking more, and find relief in doing drugs. This is only a temporary relief, not a solution, and will not help you in the long run. You get bouts of depression, don't sleep well at night, you overreact at minor annoyances, and lack concentration.

Caregiving is emotionally stressful and may cause you to go into a state of depression. For caregivers, it usually happens when we don't practice self-care and will go away if we take the time to do what we enjoy for an hour a day. The depression only lasts for a few days or maybe a few weeks. You find it hard to focus, sleep patterns change, bouts of anger, or even irritability. There were times I was so depressed I thought of suicide, I didn't want to deal with anything or anyone. These thoughts can be avoided if you know about them. Talk to your doctor.

You may develop chronic illnesses by being under too much stress. They are curable and/or preventable. In my case I developed type II diabetes and high blood pressure. My diabetes got worse over the period of fourteen years but it reversed itself a few years later and I am no longer diabetic. I am still borderline diabetic and have to be careful what I do and eat but I feel better today by doing the right things for myself.

In some cases of depression, you may have to seek help from a family doctor. Make sure the medication for depression does not affect the pills you are already taking. Your doctor will know which medications you can take.

You'll find you catch the common cold or flu more often because your body's immune system is affected with burnout. I know, near the end of my caregiving days, I was sick with a cold or flu for the entire year. I caught one thing after another.

Reach out to your friends and family, you will gain strength and energy by being with people you love and who love you back. They don't judge you and will not blame you for your feelings. Start a daily journal, sometimes just writing it down will relieve some of the pressure when you see it written down on paper. Find an activity you can do on a daily basis, even if it's a short walk outside.

Don't dwell on the things you have no control over. Your loved one isn't to blame and don't focus on how unfair life is being to you. Look for things that can make you happy and content instead. Caregiving can take over your entire life and make you miserable and sick. It happens to the best of us even when we think it won't happen, it still can.

Take one day at a time. Don't try to make matters worse by thinking ahead about what could go wrong or what you might have to do. Stay focused on the present and not on the future. It will take some time to start feeling better, just take one day at a time. You will start to replace the negative feelings with positive ones, it won't happen overnight, but you will notice the change if you take it one day at a time.

Self-care is the most important thing to do so you don't experience burnout, as I talked about it in this book. With all things, caregiver's burnout can be avoided. Learn to relax and look after yourself.

6 CARE-GIVER VERSUS WIFE AND DAUGHTER

Over the years I became a caregiver, housekeeper, cook, and part-time nurse for everyone. I had distanced myself from everyone, even my daughter and my friend. I didn't relax and would not let my guard down because if I did, I felt I would fall apart. I became a control freak with every aspect of my life and theirs. No one could do anything without me being there. I had lost myself and who I was before caregiving started. Caregiving had taken over every aspect of my life. The only thoughts I had was what I had to do next for everyone else.

With this new problem, I realized I needed to relax and let my loved ones do things for themselves and not hover over them. I treated my parents like they were my children but they never minded and my mother does not care that I am the daughter, she still likes me being in charge and I doubt that will ever change. Some people don't' like being fussed over all the time, as is the case with my husband but my mother enjoys it.

I could give up my total control of everything and everyone around me. This was something I could fix. It was hard at the start but I learned to relax and stop hovering over my husband and telling him what he could or couldn't do and just trust him that he would do the right thing and not overdo it.

I dd not realize it until many years later that I was not being a wife to my husband. I lost who I was and never knew it. My husband brought it up near the end of my caregiving days. He mentioned we were no longer as close as we once were. There was no spontaneous hug or kiss and we didn't hold hands like we used to. It was an eye opener for me. We used to be loving towards each other and I was the one who had changed and I didn't see it until it was pointed out to me. We became more like roommates, rather than husband and wife. We were two strangers that lived in the same house. It was hard to admit to myself that this was the situation at hand, and I needed to fix it. At first, I was angry at my husband for saying it, because I wouldn't have changed and lost that part of me, Afterall he was the one that got sick and created the situation in the first place.

I started to say 'I love you' again, give him a hug, call him 'Honey', or a peck on the cheek. I forgot to say it a lot of times but the more I said it, I began to remember to say it more often. When we went for a walk, I would hold his hand like we did before. Hugs and kind words were given more often and soon we became as close as we were and even closer, before this all happened.

My husband is reveling in the fact I am no longer the caregiver in the ways I used to be. We have become close and loving once again. My husband has said he can go to the family doctor by himself now. There were a few times I let him go on his own but the result was not good. The medications were wrong or missing even though I sent him with a list of his pills. He never checked the doctor's prescription and what was included. It took a while but now he can go by himself. He feels more independent now and doesn't feel like a child that needs looking after all of the time. He still talks to me if he isn't feeling good or he feels that something physically is wrong and I deal with it. Usually, when this happens, it means another visit to the family doctor.

I'm still in charge of making doctor's appointments and getting the prescriptions on time but that doesn't take much doing over the course of the year.

Along the way I found articles about what happens when a wife looks after her husband who is sick. It's a great read to find out you are not the only one out there when you find you stopped being a wife. The changes in you happen subtly and you don't even notice it when it is happening.   Be aware of it and don't dismiss the statement when people tell you that you changed and sometimes it's not for the better.

Keep an open mind and don't' react until you have had the chance to think about what was said to you. Friends and family are usually the first to see the changes in you and for the most part, are generally right. It's up to you to take it with a grain of salt and analyze it.

Only you can change yourself and make things better for you and everyone around you because if you don't, life will be harder than it has to be for you and your loved one.

7 MY FOURTEEN YEAR JOURNEY

This is the story about me as a caregiver.

I have been a caregiver for the last fourteen years and this is my journey.

No one talks about what the caregiver goes through. It's as if it is taboo to say anything about what you feel and the issues you have to deal with personally.

Caregivers are very special people and are very rare. It is one of the most difficult jobs to do. We are allowed to feel whatever we feel at the time, no matter what anyone says. I learned to embrace the feelings and accept them. Own them. This is what makes you a good caregiver. Don't get me wrong there are good days, but in the beginning, they are few and far between.

I did not have any background training from the medical profession and I was an unpaid caregiver for my family. I received no outside help and no stipend for all my efforts in caring for them. I did it because I loved them. They were my main focus but I lost myself and who I was over the years. I felt guilty for my feelings and I shouldn't have, it's a normal reaction.

I was a caregiver for my husband, my father, and I continue to be a caregiver for my mother. The load of my being a caregiver has lessened. My husband is now doing great and my father has since passed away. I am still looking after my mother, today, but it doesn't take up most of my time.

I found it hard to switch from being a caregiver back to a wife and daughter. Everyone said I was just bossy but what I was doing was making sure they were looked after. I had problems switching between caregiver and wife. Everything my husband did I would go behind him and make sure he was okay. It was hard to leave him to his own devices and I was being a mother hen instead of his wife.

The doctors and nurses I met along the way would ask me if I was in the medical profession because I seemed to have a good understanding of what was going on with the people I loved. I spent a great amount of time researching whatever was happening to them at the time, so that I could better understand what they were going through in hopes of helping my loved one's cope better.

It was a very difficult journey and sometimes I could not imagine my life being any different than it was. Being a caregiver seemed to be my lot in life and I would be doing it forever. I was grateful for the fact that my husband and my father alternated when they were sick. I don't think I could have handled it if they were sick at the same time.

I went through many changes during the years because of what was required of me being a full-time caregiver. I often thought being a caregiver full time would never end (and technically it hasn't), but some of the need has abated, and I have become better at managing my time and my caregiving activities, so I now have more time to pursue the things I want to do.

I still stay at home because my mother forgets to turn off the stove, lets things boil over, leaves the fridge door open, and breaks things. I believe she has the onset of dementia. I cannot trust her to stay at home alone. She still cooks some of the things she likes to eat but it is very seldom and when she does there is always a problem. I often need to scrub the stove when she cooks because something has boiled over, or check the taps to see if she hasn't left them running. Most times she walks away from whatever she is doing and forgets that she was in the middle of something and just goes and sits down. I'm afraid if I leave her alone, she will burn the house down. She is fully functional besides her forgetfulness and can still drive, and for the most part she can look after herself. She has high blood pressure and arthritis so there isn't much for me to do in that respect. She still wants some independence and that's ok by me, for as long as she wants it.

There are days I look back and cannot imagine all the things I went through and still be sane today, but I survived and look forward to a great future. So, I thought maybe a book about what I went through would be useful to anybody who is going through it now. It does end. Always remember: you are not alone.

So, let's begin the journey together.

8 YEAR ONE – THE YEAR MY LIFE CHANGED

In 2002, my husband and I were small business owners and our daughter was out living on her own. We had a great future ahead of us. We were bicycling, walking, and motorcycling together. It was wonderful. Nothing could stop us. We spent a lot of time together and enjoyed each other's company.

On February, 2nd, 2002, my life changed. My husband was laying on the floor in the bathroom and calling for me. It took me awhile to hear him because I was fast asleep. At first, I didn't believe him, that he had a problem, but after a few minutes I realized I had to call 911. He was having a heart attack. It was the scariest moment in my life.

The next morning, he was supposed to be installing a computer at a client's place of business and I was at a loss, I had no idea how to do that, nor was I willing to, because I needed to be by my husband's side. The doctors told me they had no idea if he was going to survive, or if his heart would give out. I ended up calling the client and explaining the situation and they were willing to wait, so, that was good.

He remained in the hospital for ten days and I was told he suffered a massive heart attack and it would take him a very long time to recover but he most likely would never be able to do the things he used to do. The hospital told me they would give me a pamphlet on do's and don'ts when I took him home. I'm not sure I would classify a two-hundred-page book a pamphlet, but that's what they called it, so, while he was in the hospital, I had time to start reading it when I was home alone.

Now came the big day and I could bring him home. I wasn't sure if I was excited, terrified, or worried.

My emotions were all over the place. I wanted him home but I didn't want to go through the ordeal again of calling 911. It wasn't made clear to me if he was out of the woods at that time.

One of the first things in my Recovery Book from the hospital, was about company coming over, only one visitor at a time and only one person a day for ten to fifteen minutes. Friends and family really wanted to see him but I had to put my foot down because I noticed he was exhausted even for that short period of time and never mind that I was too. It was hard for everyone to understand why they couldn't stay because none of us had gone through this, so, I would tell them it was time for them to leave. They always went away hurt because to them he looked fine, but I could see my husband was tired. My husband did not want them to see him as weak, but I could tell, and everyone thought I was being over-protective. I wasn't, I knew my husband and could tell when he just wanted to be alone. Our friends did not understand and wanted to stay longer, sometimes they would stay five or ten minutes longer and Hubbie would fall asleep. I wanted to talk to my best friend about what I was going through but Hubbie was with me all the time, so, I just stayed quiet. Keeping things internally was absolutely not beneficial to me.

I hated what was happening, all the pressure that was put on me, and I hated my life, my husband, and everything around me. I even hated myself for feeling like that, but it wasn't anyone's fault, so, I struggled to keep my spirits up. I always loved candles and would light up a bunch of them and it somehow helped.

I know now that I need to express my emotions, or purge them. Sometimes exercise works. Sometimes painting, or learning a new language, or soaking in a bath, reading, or even doing a crossword puzzle helps, but I didn't know that then, and I suffered more than I needed to. There are many health chapters in your area, that will help. I did not have that then, nor did I ever think of it. Look online, I'm sure there are some in your area. I have just become aware of a 24/7 healthlink hotline in our area, staffed with medical practitioners capable of addressing my concerns, that wasn't available at the time, whom I could talk to without leaving my husband alone. I could have called when he was asleep.

Each of us will go through a different crisis because of the situation with our loved ones, but I want to share with you what I did. The recovery book I got gave me guidelines and I found them to be very useful. I'm sure your situation will be different, but nonetheless, use the information given to you by the medical sector, they have been doing it for a long time and offer great advice.

My recovery book stated he had to go for a walk every day to strengthen his heart. Granted, it was only a few hundred feet for the first few weeks, but he had to walk. Now for the part I found humorous – 'he was not allowed to walk into the wind.' Uh, how does one do that exactly? Suppose we started our walk when it was calm, and then a wind hustled up? I couldn't just leave him there, standing on the sidewalk while I went home to get the vehicle, because he was not about to stay there by himself, and I don't know if it was possible to go out when it wasn't windy. It was quite a conundrum for me, so we went anyway, but the walk took longer when we were walking into the wind.

I took over our business and things got very difficult for me. I learned all the things he did with the business. I knew my side, accounting, web design, and programming. I was so nervous when I installed a computer onsite and setup their network, that I didn't sleep the night before. In the morning I put on a brave face and no one could see what I was going through. I didn't want the client to see me insecure so I wanted to look like I knew what I was doing but I hadn't a clue. I thought I would be going by myself but my husband would not stay home by himself so I took him with me. Ah, moral support! My husband was exhausted by the time we got there and could not stay awake. So, while I did the work, he dozed in the chair. I suggested he might be more comfortable taking a nap in the car but he wouldn't sit there by himself, so he just stayed close to me. The job got done and I was proud of myself, I did it and still managed to look after my husband. That was the beginning of my life changing for the better.

I would get home in the evening and cook and clean and make sure Hubbie was resting ok. I went with him to all his doctors' appointments and sat in with the doctor to tell him how Hubbie was doing because when asked the question, 'How are you doing?', Hubbie would always say he was "good, nothing wrong". But Hubbie always told me what was going on with him so I made sure I told the doctor how he was doing, how he was feeling, and what hurt, and what he was able to do or not do.

By the second week I was totally exhausted. Weekends consisted of cleaning the house and shoveling snow, and it snowed a lot that year. I was definitely getting my exercise. It felt like I was running on fumes. I found myself crying and feeling sorry for myself because I could not get a moment alone or sit down for five minutes.

I was exhausted and burnt out. I had no time for myself, and with work and home, I had no time for emotions or feeling sorry for myself. I felt I had no choice but to keep going. I didn't sleep well at night, always listening to make sure Hubbie was still breathing. In a way, it was a blessing that I was exhausted, I didn't feel anything, I kept going.

I started getting sick, I became diabetic, high blood pressure, run down. Now I made sure we were both taking our pills. His were different times than mine, so, it seemed all I was doing was distributing medications all day and evening long. I bought a pill box and a pill cutter from the pharmacy to fill up once a month. It became much easier to keep track of them at that point.

I wanted to join a support group after the first week but Hubbie said I didn't need that, and besides, he wasn't about to sit at home by himself. A support group was off the table for me and I just couldn't think straight at the time. Now there are so many support sites online, and a host of services available like Skip the Dishes, (oh that would have been nice), cleaning services, which I did not think of either. A baby monitor would have been helpful, I wouldn't have to walk to the bedroom so many times to check on him and could have cleaned the house quicker, or soaked in the tub longer if only I would have had one.

My family doctor noted that I wasn't looking well and I explained what I was feeling and going through. She told me that I had better smarten up because, "who would look after my husband if something happened to me?" I never looked at it that way. At this point I realized I needed to make some changes so I could look after myself better. She was a firm believer that less medications, not more was better, and if she prescribed a pill for depression, chances were that it would affect the diabetes pills I was on. Had I not become diabetic I probably would have gotten an anti-depression medication. It might have helped.

I finally started to lock myself in the bathroom for ten minutes, have a good cry and carry on. Hubbie never knew what I was going through and never saw me cry, because he was going through something worse than I was. It would make him feel guilty, on top of everything else, knowing I was crying and I didn't want him to see me like that. I felt like my life was unbearable, it was impossible for me to see that it would get better again, so I went through the motions and carried on. Today, it is better and I can do the things I like to do and we are both enjoying life again but back then I did not see any hope for the future. I was scared. I only concentrated on one day at a time. I read through the recovery book on the things

Hubbie was allowed to do because I wanted his recovery to go well.

I wanted my husband back the way he used to be but I could see the change in him. He was angry, afraid, and felt guilty for what happened. It wasn't his fault that he had a heart attack but I couldn't convince him of that. I took him to see the cardiologist every week for the first three months which took at least two to three hours out of that day. I scheduled appointments for the business around those days so I learned to fix the problems our clients had more efficiently so I could deal with Hubbie and his issues. It felt like time was against us. Time for doctors, time for clients, time for taking care of Hubbie, time for domestic duties, and no time just for me.

I didn't involve our daughter in any of this because she was entitled to have a life of her own and besides, she was working, living on her own, and going to University as well. I did not need to burden her any more than she already was.

I did it on my own but I had expected my mother to help, after all, she is my mother, but she never did. She only wanted me to help them on top of what I was going through with my husband. My life had become a nightmare and I could not see a way out.

Prior to his heart attack, Hubbie had never learned to cook, but it was something he was supposed to do, according to the book, so with my help, he began making soup. He found he really liked chopping vegetables but had no idea what to do with them. I stayed by his side and told him how to make soup. Somehow chopping veggies was very soothing for him, so every Saturday, I let him cook. I kept an eye on him making sure he didn't cut off a thumb or finger because he was quite unbalanced and a bit clumsy. I guess lack of oxygen to your brain does that to a person. This did not free up any of my time but he was beginning to feel better about himself and didn't feel so useless anymore. He was now contributing and thought it was one less thing on my plate. It wasn't because I still watched over him and then I cleaned the kitchen afterwards. But it was worth it to see him gain some independence and confidence. He was trying to do things for himself and he began pushing his limits to find out if he could do more.

Almost a month had passed since the day of his heart attack and he was able to walk around the block. When we got home, he was exhausted and needed to lie down, so I would check on him every few minutes to see if he was still breathing. I was starting to get used to my new way of life as a caregiver. I wasn't as angry anymore, or afraid, or frustrated. This was the way life was going to be, so, I adapted to the new lifestyle. I still had a good cry every now and then but it wasn't as often anymore.

Our daughter would visit every weekend and she would make me laugh. It was a good sign if I found something funny, it meant I was getting better. After she went home, I found myself laughing at whatever she had said or done, for days after. I felt better after laughing and now I also began my road to recovery. It was painstakingly slow but maybe, just maybe, I thought, life would get better. There were days I think people would have said I had gone crazy, because I would sit in the kitchen by myself and start laughing for a while remembering something funny.

After three months, Hubbie was able to help at work, granted not for a very long period of time, but it was something, a beginning for him. As he began to feel better, so did I.

His cardiologist said that he was doing better than expected and I was to keep doing whatever I was doing because it was working. Yay me!

Work, house, snow, and anything thing else in life seemed a little lighter and not so hopeless anymore. Friends could visit a bit longer, which helped me. My best friend of thirty years would come over and cheer me up.

My daughter made me laugh. I wasn't as depressed as I was for the past month and there was hope for a better future. Having a support system, people who care about you as much as they care about your loved one, can make a huge difference in how your journey unfolds.

I had lost my husband of old but I gained a new one because he had changed. He was very different now but it didn't matter as long as he was still with me.

Whatever I was going through, he was going through it worse, so if he could work through it, so would I. So, I put on my big girl pants and started enjoying life and dealing with everything that came my way without feeling sorry for myself and being angry or depressed. He was amazing, he was fighting to get back, and he inspired me. It was a difficult period in my life but watching him trying to get better made me rethink things about me. It made me stronger and able to cope with everything much better.

I had a new and different husband and a new way of life. I gained a career and was now a contributing partner in the business and felt great about myself. I realized I had also changed. Life was now looking better and a bit cheerier. As I began to feel better about myself, I noticed, Hubbie began to feel better too. Whatever I was doing as a caregiver, it was working for both of us. We were never apart, we spent 24-7 together. I truly enjoyed that now because I didn't have to be looking after him all the time. Rather than a mother hen looking after her chick, I could discover the new person he was becoming and I could enjoy his company. He was no longer a full-time burden. I never tired of him and reveled in the fact we could spend every minute together and never wanted to be apart.

Today, fourteen years later, he goes to work by himself. I find I miss him when he's gone. I look forward to retirement when we can be together all the time.

Six months after that horrible event he needed to

start driving. It was pretty evident he was still out of sorts and didn't have much focus while driving but I let him try to do it anyway. He got better every day but he got exhausted by just driving. I really didn't need this. I was just getting used to my new life but he needed to gain more independence, so I let him drive. It was quite terrifying and I wished I had my own brake installed in the vehicle, but I did not. By the end of the first year he was doing much better.

I got into a rhythm and didn't feel as stressed or tired as I used to be, so everything was going well.

By the end of one year we were both doing well and I was enjoying life again. It wasn't as hard, I had a sense of humor again, I was laughing, and having fun. It is true what they say, laughter is the best medicine. The event now seemed like a lifetime away and getting further away every day.

I regret not using the resources at the time available to me. It would have made it much easier to deal with if I could have talked to someone about what I was going through.

Emotions of the Year – Working Pages

That year the strongest emotions I had were: hatred, annoyed, anxious, sad, and hopeless.

Do you feel hatred?

You are entitled you your feelings, no matter what they are. It is you and only you who knows how hard it is to be a caregiver. I didn't know much about the internet at the time but there are so many resources out there, use them. You don't have to feel that you are alone in this. You have a right to have feelings and emotions, don't let anyone make you believe otherwise.

I feel hatred because:

_____

Do you feel annoyed?

I found myself snapping at people for no reason, and then I would feel guilty about it, especially when they didn't deserve it. Everybody seemed happy, I was not. I remember once I was standing in line at a self-checkout and a person didn't know how to use it and the girl working there was helping this person ring through all her items and I blew up at them. I had an item that wouldn't scan and I wanted help too. I had no patience then. Afterwards I felt horrible. Making a conscious effort to be kind to people around me was hard but in the end it worked. I didn't feel as bad because I wasn't being mean to anyone.

I feel annoyed because:

_____

Do you feel anxious?

I found I had anxiety problems, my heart would race, or it was erratic, and most times I was out of breath, for no reason. There were many times I found if I sat down and tried to control my breathing by slowly breathing in and out, it would help.

I feel anxious because:

_____

Do you feel sad?

There were times when I was just sad. I felt life had thrown me under the bus. How could I feel better when all I looked forward to was this? I thought it would never end. I thought I would never be able to do things I wanted to do ever again. But it did end, or, at least, it got easier. I just couldn't see it then. I would sometimes step outside and try to see the beauty in the world. It was quite difficult, but sometimes just noticing a butterfly or bird would lighten my spirit. There are so many good things to see if we only try to look.

I feel sad because:

Do you feel hopeless?

It all seemed hopeless to me, being a caregiver, and for what? Why did this happen to me? I wasn't the one that got sick, yet I felt I was being punished by live. But life has a way of going on even if you don't want it to. Watching my husband struggle every day was hard, but seeing what he was going through, I realized my life was much easier. He was trying to gain back his independence and I was feeling sorry for myself.

I feel hopeless because:

Tips from the Trenches

(TIP) Don't try to do everything yourself. Talk to someone. Check out what's available for you online.

(TIP) Cherish the good days, there will be a few in the beginning but as you go along there will be many more to come. Remember those days!

(TIP) Treat yourself to your favorite beverage or food. It will give you a short time-out.

 (TIP) Phone or text a friend. They are always ready to listen and help and even if they don't, talking to someone that isn't going through what you are, helps.

(TIP) Anger produces energy. You can use that energy towards something constructive until it runs out.

(TIP) Try some deep-breathing exercises for a few minutes.

(TIP) Take a five-minute walk outside.

(TIP) A little planning goes a long way. Whether it is a pill box to organize meds for a week or more at a time, or making large batches of food to save on needing to cook every day, little bits of planning can buy you the time you need to not only care effectively for your loved one, but also to get a few moments to care for yourself.

(TIP) Ask for help. Often, people don't know what to

do to help. But if you ask them to bring a meal, or do the grocery shop, or help spell you from watching over your loved one, you will be surprised at how often the answer is "yes, I would be happy to do that for you".

What I learned about myself…

Looking back at the year, we noticed a change in both of us. I was now strong and able to do anything life had to throw at me. There were still a lot of bad days but even through those days, I changed. I could cope with anything. On a daily basis, I never saw me changing but by the end of the year, I had.

I became confident in what I was doing, workwise. I was no longer as shy as I was before this year. I saw changes in me that were for the better. I always worked by myself prior to this year. I did, bookkeeping, web pages, and programming in Access, so, dealing with people wasn't what I had to do. Now I was able to talk to people with confidence and I enjoyed it.

I discovered I was very good at being a caregiver, even the doctors were telling me that. I never knew I had it in me before.

I did not know I could go through a major crisis and come out the other side being better than I was before the event. Even though all the bad emotions were there, I still managed to look at the good side. We were learning to cope with these changes to our lives, and began the healing process. I was taking life one day at a time and before I knew it a year had gone by.

On the Lighter Side…

My daughter was living in an apartment complex and decided that she wanted to move from the basement to the third floor. My husband would not be able to help much because the lifting and carrying restrictions on him did not allow him to carry anything over five kilograms.

I knew he was going to push it but I told my

daughter she would have to get some strong guys to do the majority of the lifting. She got a few men from work to help. We were all enjoying ourselves, a bit tired from doing all the stairs, (her apartment did not have an elevator), but nonetheless, we were having fun but I kept an eye on my husband because he wouldn't admit to his weakness at the time and would pick up boxes that contained her books. Those boxes were the heaviest and he was bound and determined he could carry them. We removed the boxes from him and gave him lighter ones. He thought he was just as strong as before his heart attack.

The men were told at the beginning that my husband was not allowed to carry anything heavy and they were quite good at keeping the heavy stuff away from her Dad but my husband kept pushing it until I told him we were going to go and get pizza and beer for the boys, this way he could not get into any more trouble.

The guys were amazing. They never complained, and never got tired of doing all the lifting and carrying up the stairs. While we were gone one of the boys looked over to my daughter and said, "Is that Alex's boyfriend?"

My daughter's response was, "Sort of, that's my mom, and that's my dad".

When they had gone my daughter told us the story and we all laughed. "I didn't hire them for their brains, I hired them for their brawn," she exclaimed.

9 YEAR TWO – MAKING EXERCISE FUN

The second year had new challenges. The whole exercising thing, walking, was exhausting. Instead of driving everywhere, we walked. We would walk to the mall near us and pick up groceries and carry them home. Needless to say, we did not buy much, because they became heavy after a while and he was not allowed to carry anything over a certain weight, so I carried the bulk of it. I became a pack mule. I remember one time that year when I saw a picture of a woman pulling a cart and her husband sitting in it and the caption wrote, "husband of the year award." I couldn't stop laughing because that was me. That year I looked around to see if I could get him a trophy that had that caption and I did get one engraved. Needless to say, he was not amused but I found it very funny. Still today there are times when he realizes I did something that he should have done and he looks at me and says, "Yup, I get husband of the year award, again."

The more we walked, the more we could walk and we could now walk all day. The second year I got tired of walking twenty-five kilometers a day, so, we took up bicycling during the summer. We started out slowly, around the block for the first while and gradually increasing the distance. I always enjoyed riding a bike, so it was a treat. We would bicycle to the mall and get a few groceries and come home. Then we started going a bit further. Now we would ride to our clients' place of business, (they thought we were crazy), do what was required, and carried on. I was truly enjoying my life. It was different but somehow better than it was before his heart attack. We were spending quality time together, it was wonderful. One time while we were biking, one of our client's noticed us and began honking. Scared the life out of me but when they pulled up along-side of us, we realized who they were and they were smiling and waving at us. I would rather have gotten a thumbs up sign because I'm not sure if they were smiling or laughing at us. That year we found out one of our client's had suffered a stroke and a heart attack. We got to compare stories and found out that he and my husband went through similar things. I think that's when I realized I wasn't the only one going through this.

It's funny how an event like that can change your life for the better if you want it to. I know it was still hard on my husband but each day he would get stronger. He was still angry and depressed because as he said, "The Grim Reaper knows his name", all he meant by that was he now knew he would die one day. I didn't want to hear that. When you're in your forties, I don't think anyone thinks that or believes it, but there it was. I was only forty-three when I almost became a widow and realized that death was inevitable and one day, I would be alone, without him. It was always at the back of my mind. It still is but I don't dwell on it as much anymore.

We started riding our bikes downtown to look around, have lunch, join in the summer festivities that were there when we didn't have any calls to go on. Summer was nice, we could be outside, enjoy the days. Putting seventy kilometers on our bikes was a normal day for us and we both had the stamina to do it. We were now frequenting book stores on our bicycles throughout the city and it was a lot of fun. We ended up buying saddlebags for our bikes to carry stuff we bought. In August we have Heritage days and the Fringe. We never went to the events before because there is no place to park, but on our bicycles, it wasn't a problem. So, now we could find out what those events were all about. We even had our daughter going with us. She was able to be with her Dad and get to know him after he had changed because when she came over to visit, her Dad was always resting in bed. She didn't know how different he had become but he could now give out one-liner jokes that were hilarious to us because before his heart attack, he was not funny and couldn't tell a joke for the life of him and now all of a sudden, he could. He didn't see what was so funny when he said something, so we would explain it to him.

I think the one thing you have to do, is find something you have in common with your loved one and focus on that. Encourage them, guide them, and push them to do things even if they don't want to. They can't get better if they just sit at home and mope and that was my job and so I did it. Hubbie did not need much pushing, he was always a doer but every now and then, it was harder.

We both had our motorcycle licenses, but I was reluctant to let him get on his motorcycle because of his lack of focus. His driving ability was poor, and on a motorcycle, you need a lot more focus than driving a car. I knew I was going to let him try but I was hesitant. He finally convinced me that he was capable and so we went for our first ride in years. He had no attention span and almost ran into the back of a car, so, he now realized he was not ready for that. It was one less thing for me to worry about. I was relieved.

We were both avid readers but after his heart attack he wasn't able to read, that part of his brain was damaged. He kept trying to read. I saw him struggle with it and he just kept at it. He was never one to quit, so, slowly he was making progress. By the end of the second year, he was able to get through a book. I was getting enough time that I could read when I wanted to and I was doing great. I got my life back to some extent.

Winter has always been six to seven months long here, so, I shoveled snow a lot. Hubbie was never allowed to shovel snow again. Great!!! I wanted to get a snow-blower but Hubbie wouldn't let me. He said, "If you get a snow-blower I will lose hope in the fact I will never be allowed to shovel snow". I'm pretty sure the doctors told me he could never shovel ever again because there was the possibility that his heart could stop. I was annoyed with Hubbie. No snow-blower for me in the near future, shoveling it was, but if it was a self-propelled one, he could have been in charge of the snow, but I could not explain it to him. He would not hear me. He felt bad that he couldn't help me and so he got angry, not at me, but at himself for getting sick. I dealt with his anger. That was hard because before his heart attack, he was not an angry person, he had a big heart, and never got upset. This was out of character for him and I wasn't sure how to deal with it. Something new for me to learn about him and how to accept this behavior. He was so different now his personality had changed.

We walked during the winter even when it was minus forty degrees Celsius. I did not enjoy the cold but I did it anyway. He didn't want to walk in the malls, I never understood why and even to this day I don't. He couldn't walk very far because of the weather and the deepness of the snow, it made him tired but we still did it to the best of his ability.

In the recovery book, it said, he should learn a new language or take up playing a musical instrument. I have played music since the age of five and I could help him. I could explain music terminology and teach him. This did not help me gain more time for myself but I saw him change and get better. He could focus longer and was doing much better. It helped him because he became less angry and I could see he was a little happier. He mentioned to me when we first got married that he wanted to play a musical instrument but never got the opportunity. Now was his chance to learn. He never realized how hard it is to learn but he soon discovered what it took. He had always told me I had the gift, it is not a gift, it's how much time and effort you put into it.

I enrolled him in music lessons because he stopped listening to me and I also thought that this would be a great opportunity to get some time for myself while he was in his lesson, but he said he wanted me to sit in on the lessons. This kind of defeated the purpose of me getting a half hour by myself. I encouraged him to try one lesson on his own and he agreed. It went well. I was off the clock as a caregiver, even if it was very short, it was nice.

It was pointless for me to go home for half an hour so I hung out at the music store. I enjoyed it a lot, I could browse through the music books and check out the instruments. It was amazing how fast a half hour flew by but now I could relax even if it was a half hour. Sometimes I would go next door to the coffee shop and wait. I got to meet a lot of nice people. I wasn't as isolated as before. I wasn't as shy as I was and I began striking up conversation with total strangers. I met a lady who also had a husband that suffered a stroke, she said it was hard, we got to compare stories, and found out it's all the same no matter what the illness is, we went through similar things being a caregiver.

I also found out about a client of ours that had a stroke first and a couple of years later suffered a heart attack. He was going through the same things my husband was at the time. They compared stories and I would do the work but I could listen in to what they were saying. He became a social butterfly. He would chat with anyone and that was out of character for him, he never liked idle chit chat before. I was glad he could talk to other people now and not just me.

By the end of the second year my husband still had bouts of depression and anger but I didn't spend too much time dwelling on that but told him about all the things he was able to do now, it helped him and it also helped me. I was gaining more time for me which in turn made me feel better. It was still hard but the fear of losing him was disappearing from my mind and there were more better days than worse.

Emotions of the Year – Working Pages

That year the strongest emotions I had were: feeling worse, better, happy, lost, and drained.

Do you feel worse?

There were days I felt like I was getting worse, not better. I was lethargic, lazy, and just not wanting to be alive anymore. Most of the days were good, some were even great, but other days, and there weren't that many, I would feel worse. I realized it depended on what my husband was feeling and began watching out that I didn't feel the same. I'm a very empathetic person, when someone is happy, I am too. I needed to know if it was me or my husband that was angry, depressed, or even sad. I found out it was mostly him, so I made an effort instead to cheer him up and bring him out of that mood.

I feel worse because:

_____

Do you feel better?

Some days I felt I was on top of the world and I got to enjoy every minute of it but I still watched out for what my husband was feeling so I wouldn't fall into that trap. It was as if we had become one person, what he felt, I felt.

I feel better because:

_____

Do you feel happy?

I found that I was feeling happy a lot of the times and when that happened, I let myself be happy.

I feel happy because:

_____

Do you feel lost?

As my husband gained more of his independence back, I felt lost. I didn't know what to do with myself and began exploring some hobbies that would amuse me. Now, there I was getting what I asked for and finding out I don't know what to do myself. I felt useless, nobody needed me, and I had all the time in the world now, what conflicting thoughts those were. On one hand I wanted to be able to do what I wanted and on the other hand I felt empty now.

I feel lost because:

_____

Do you feel drained?

Some days I felt completely drained. It usually happened when I took my husband to his cardiologist at the hospital. Four hours were lost out of the day because of waiting. By the time we got home I was completely drained. Taking a bath or shower that was almost too hot made me feel better.

I feel drained because:

_____

Tips from the Trenches

(TIP) Taking a hot shower or bath will drain the tension out of your body and help you relax. If you like baths use Epsom salts or scented bubble bath.

(TIP) Enjoy a hobby if you have one. It doesn't matter how long you get to do it, but it does relax the mind doing something you like.

(TIP) When you're waiting at the pharmacy for medications, check out their pamphlets, there is a lot of information for caregivers.

What I learned about myself…

I began to enjoy bicycling and walking. I never liked outside activities before but now it seemed different. I started looking forward to it each and every day. I started liking the thought of being in the great outdoors.

They say misery loves company but just knowing there were other people out there that were also going through something, let me realize we weren't the only ones going through an event, before this, I felt isolated. I only saw what we were going through and that was my mistake. I started to open up to people and talk to them.

I was growing and changing every day and started getting excited to see what the changes would be in the future. By the end of each year I could stop and assess what the changes were, even my personality was changing. I was an outgoing, confident person. People actually enjoyed being with me and talking to me, that was just so weird. I never had many friends while growing up and now I had people on my side ready to help or just be there. I wasn't alone anymore and that was a nice feeling.

On the Lighter Side…

We went to Heritage Days on our bicycles, there is o parking available for vehicles, and I was looking forward to tasting all the international foods there. We locked up our bikes and began sampling food we never tried before.

I remember I wanted to try the Rose Tea. Oh, how awful that was. It truly tasted like a rose, not that I ever ate a rose leaf, but it did taste like a rose. Yuck! I promptly threw it away. Some of the foods are good and some are really horrible but you never know until you try it.

We were enjoying the taste experience and it was a nice sunny, warm, Saturday. It was our first time at this event and didn't know what to expect. There were stage shows of all sorts and we watched them perform, some of them were spectacular.

My husband is of Swedish descent and we came across a booth that had Swedish food. There was a dessert that was called 'leftsa', we got my daughter one and while she's eating it my husband looks over and says, "is it as a good as a 'rightsa'.

46

I was taking a sip of my beverage at the time and choked on it because it was just so unexpected of my husband to be funny.

Oh, great, now my husband had become a comedian. He could shoot off one-liners that would make everyone laugh. He went from being serious and never being able to tell a joke, to being the funniest guy ever.

10 YEAR THREE – SQUIRREL STEALING MY TOAST

The third year was amazing. My husband was feeling more confident about himself and he was now happy. I was happier because he was beginning to do things for himself and he didn't need me as much. I had more time for me. He had changed and I felt like I had married someone else, he was so different. He kept telling me he wanted to get back to his old self, I don't think he actually remembered who he was before.

At the start of the third year, I was feeling good about myself, I helped my husband through his ordeal and realized I had become an amazing person. Once a week we made time to play pool at a billiards hall and also try our hand at karaoke. When we played pool, he would hit the balls so hard they would fly off the table. I was told by my husband to stand in front of the balls he was going to shoot at so I would stop them from flying into other people and so I did. I should have brought along a goalie's outfit because it was impossible to catch the balls and even if I could have it would have hurt. I was really bad at playing pool but he didn't mind, it was all about being together and having fun. We had never tried singing but we wanted to see what it was like. So, the first time we tried, the chorus came up and my husband looked at me and asked, "What language is that?" I laughed because it was just something like, "wee dee dee", you get the idea. He was still having difficulty reading and I didn't realize it but we even got a certificate that day for trying and I still have it today.

His driving ability had improved greatly and he could go by himself, so I felt confident we could start riding our motorcycles. As time went on, we went on day excursions and visited some small towns in the area. We decided we should take some time off but my husband never liked to taking holidays. I brought up the idea to take a week off and go to the mountains but we would take our bikes instead of a vehicle. He jumped at the chance and we got on our bikes and grabbed two sleeping bags, a tent, and two backpacks. The backpacks contained sundry items, clothes, a camping stove, and all his medications.

When we arrived at the camp ground, they put us in a section with other motorcyclists. We met really nice people that week. The whole time we were there it rained but I didn't mind. We would walk to town and back every day. We would see the sights, get our food and go to our campsite and cook up what we brought back. We were always exhausted by the time we got back but it made us sleep better. We kept our food locked up because of the bears but every morning I made toast. One time I turned my back on the toast and saw a squirrel take off with it. We were warned not to feed the wildlife and I wasn't trying to but what's to say if they steal it, so I chased him and caught him, the piece of toast was much bigger than him so it wasn't a problem, it slowed the little guy down a lot. My husband thought I would hate the trip because it rained the whole time and instead, he found out it was the best camping trip ever, for me. We felt invigorated when we got back and could take on the world together once more.

We were beginning to do things we had never done before and life was fun again. I wasn't as scared or depressed anymore and I could see us having a wonderful future together.

My life was turning around, I no longer looked after my husband as much and I had more time to myself. The dark cloud that floated above us was now lifting and we both saw a better life coming.

We started bicycling through the city parks, went everywhere on our bikes, walked every day and began to see the world differently. We didn't worry as much as we had, my husband had worried about me being ok if he died but now, he felt he would survive and he didn't have to think about that and neither did I. Things were beginning to look up and we were invincible once again.

By the end of three years he was doing well and was now ready to go back to work on his own and I now felt lost because he no longer needed me, and just like that he took back his business and I was semi-retired. He would call on me when there was a job he couldn't do. I wanted to keep working but he wanted to do the lion's share and so I had a lot of time on my hands to pursue other things.

My husband had purchased an oil painting course that I could learn because I had always wanted to learn how to paint in oils and acrylics. So, I began to paint. I wasn't very good, but that didn't matter, because I had the time and it was something new for me to try and I always liked learning and doing new things.

I have always had a lot of hobbies and now I had time to get back to them, it was great. I crocheted, cross-stitched, did puzzles of all kinds, and read books. It was a time for rest and relaxation for me and I took advantage of it. I started walking by myself and enjoyed being by myself. It was an adjustment for me not to have to look after someone else all the time. I looked after myself and learned to enjoy it. At the time I didn't realize it but nothing lasts forever so I was glad I took the time for me because it wasn't long after when my father became ill.

I was grateful for the time, it meant I could do anything I wanted so I began to cook gourmet dishes, I always enjoyed cooking, and I now had the time to make special dinners. My husband was happy that I was happy.

We still bicycled and walked but it was at the end of the day and not during. He enjoyed the new dishes I prepared, he always loved eating the food I made but these were different and they were heart smart foods.

When he started working by himself, I found I

missed my husband because we were inseparable for three years but I had to let him do things alone and stop being a mother hen. I felt more like his wife now, than his caregiver but I was still both but more a wife than anything at this point. It was the other way around before and I didn't know which I preferred at this point. I had become so accustomed to being a caregiver that it became a way of life for me and now it was gone. I still made sure he had his medications and that he took them on time. He only had two visits to the doctor's a year now and I still sat in on them. I needed to know if he really was getting better and he was.

It was a year of growth for me. I was able to enjoy my time alone, which I never liked doing before. I was glad I capitalized on the time allowed to me because a few months later my father got ill and I was back on the job as a caregiver. My mother and father always had a love-hate relationship. She in no way was ever a caregiver.

Emotions of the Year – Working Pages

That year the strongest emotions I had were: grateful, sorry, elated, good, and exhilarated.

Do you feel grateful?

I saw an amazing transformation between my husband and me. We had come a long way and we had both changed. I was grateful for getting a chance to spend so much time with my husband.

I feel grateful because:

_____

Do you feel sorry?

Both of us would sometimes get angry and say things we shouldn't have to each other but in the morning, we apologized and carried on. We always felt sorry for what we said, we just didn't think, before we spoke. Life goes on.

I feel sorry because:

_____

Do you feel elated?

There were days I felt so happy I could burst. Life was so much better than it was before and we were making progress every day with my husband getting better. I have always loved astronomy and I picked up a university course on astrophysics. It was difficult but I was doing very well at it. I was feeling good about myself and I really loved learning something new. It took up most of my days and evenings studying. I was just so pleased with myself now.

I feel elated because:

_____

Do you feel good?

Certain days I just felt good. I felt good about myself and what I had done for my husband, he was getting healthier and started to enjoy his life again, and so did I.

I feel good because:

_____

Do you feel exhilarated?

I felt exhilarated some days. I had energy to do anything and everything I wanted to do. Those days were the best days and I took advantage of them. After a visit to the cardiologist, we found out he had no damage to his heart and it made us feel we could conquer the world. Now, we could accomplish everything that we had planned before the event. We were unstoppable. It was such a good feeling.

I feel exhilarated because:

_____

Tips from the Trenches

(TIP) Strike up a conversation with a stranger and say a

kind word to them you'll be amazed how much it will make you feel better.

(TIP) Look outside at the splendor in the world around you.

(TIP) Pat yourself on the back, you deserve it. No one else will but you can definitely feel good about yourself for being an amazing caregiver.

What I learned about myself...

I was never outside for any length of time when it rained but I was enjoying it. On our camping trip, all it did was rain and instead of being miserable, I was laughing about it, relishing the adventure. I couldn't stop talking about the fun we had to anyone that would stop and listen. I put together an album with all the pictures we took and showed it to everyone. I gained confidence in my riding ability.

I was striking up conversations with complete strangers while camping which was unusual for me but I met many fascinating people and enjoyed listening to their stories. It was a wonderful time to be alive.

On the Lighter Side...

When we were at the camp-site we found the cabin where we could sit when it was raining. We were sitting inside and another couple came in.

We struck up a conversation with them. The man looked like a thug, straggly beard, long hair, and disheveled. A bit frightening at the start but talking to him we found out he was the head of the IT department at a University in Phoenix. What a surprise that was.

I now had someone to talk to that did the same things I did, programming and websites. We spent the whole afternoon shooting the breeze and exchanging stories. It turned out to be a wonderful day. Don't judge a book by its cover, is all I could think of that day.

Now the next day we went to get firewood and

there was a small bridge over a creek. It looked okay. My husband crossed it, no problem, I crossed it, problem. I did not realize the boards were not nailed down and I put my foot on the edge of a board, next thing I know, I'm lying down in the creek, soaking wet. I was not amused. My husband tried to pull me out but I was in an awkward position and I managed to drag him in to the creek with me. He was not amused but I didn't get my two cameras wet through all this because they were in my pockets.

Later that day we went back to the same bridge and noticed someone had put up a sign that read, "Please don't break our bridge." Seriously, I wasn't trying to break the bridge but don't you think you should make the bridge sturdier and fasten the boards down?

It was the best vacation I ever had even though we were wet and cold for the most part.

11 YEAR FOUR – MY SPOKE BROKE

I always saw my father as a strong independent man all my life but this time I saw him frightened and fragile. He had never spent any time in a hospital and I didn't know how he would take it.

That year my life became a nightmare. My father got ill and my mother couldn't handle it. She was never a caregiver and didn't know what it entailed, so, I took over. I didn't realize it at the time but she let him overdose on painkillers and he went into a coma and fell to the floor. My mother called me to come over and help. I told her to call 911 but she would not, in fear of them asking her a question, so I would drive over and call emergency and it all started again. My life was no longer mine again. My parents immigrated to Canada in 1958 and never bothered to learn English well enough. I was supposed to read for them, write, and explain things to them that they didn't understand my whole life.

This was the first time my mother was alone in the house at night and every sound startled her whether the noise came from inside the house or out. She would call in the middle of the night because she heard something and I would have to drive over and check around the house. She did not do well by herself at night and begged me to stay over. I refused. A lot of people live alone and don't have a problem but she always did. I did not get much sleep while my father was in hospital because she called every night. I found I was very irritable, angry, and frustrated.

I drove her to the hospital every day to visit my father because she didn't know what to do in a parking lot where you have to pay. She didn't want to learn and refused to see my father by herself. She never realized what pressure she put on me. It was up to me to do everything for her and I still made sure my husband went to his doctor's appointments, which I sat in on too.

In many ways it was harder this time because I would drive over to their place, pick her up and drive her to the hospital. It was a lot more time consuming. I didn't think it was fair to me being in this situation.

When my father was released, I took care of him and her, made sure he went to hospital and doctor's meetings, and sat in with his appointments because they didn't understand what doctors said, nor did they know their way around hospitals. I began to feel like a guide dog, I was duty bound to look after them and there was no way out of this.

Again, my father went into a self-induced coma, or, with the aid of my mother, and was hospitalized. He would slip in and out of the coma and things were not looking good. The doctors came and told me to expect the worst because his heart was now very erratic and asked if we had a DNR (Do Not Resuscitate) in place. No, we did not have one. The doctor asked my mother who was going to be responsible for the decision when the time came. She flatly refused to take on the responsibility and told them I was going to make the final decision.

So, now I found I was the person to be responsible for him living or dying. I was absolutely flabbergasted. Shouldn't she have been the one for making such a decision? They had been married for over fifty years at this point and she should decide, not me, but there it was.

I was terrified because if I made the wrong decision my mother could hate me for the rest of her life and blame me. He did eventually wake up and recover. He came home and I took all the painkillers I could find and threw them away. I did not know they had hundreds of them stashed away under their beds.

I found it more time consuming and exhausting than just looking after my husband, which I was still doing. He also still had his doctor's appointments and a cardiologist appointment once a year, which I took him to.

At this point it was becoming evident that I was going into a state of depression again. I was exhausted, frustrated and crying most of the time. Now I had three people to look after and I had no time for me. Life became unbearable again. I was constantly on the go, day and night.

After my father's stay at the hospital his family doctor discovered he had blocked arteries and we were informed he would require several stents. I had no idea what that was. I researched it and asked the doctor questions because I would have to explain it to my parents.

Because he was going to go through this procedure, we attended pre-op classes, which I made sure we did. I took him for his bloodwork, and made sure he wouldn't take certain medications before his surgery. I drove them to the hospital on time, which meant, 4:00 a.m.

When they took him in for the procedure, my mother and I went to the coffee shop on the same floor. While we were there my mother kept rambling on about nothing and got me frazzled. We went back to the room to wait for my father when I realized I forgot my purse at the coffee shop. I started to panic, all my credit cards, driver's license, and keys were in my purse. I ran back to where we were sitting and my purse was not there. I wouldn't be able to drive home and my address was on my driver license so whoever took my purse could go to my house and help themselves, after all they had my keys. Someone saw me and asked if I had lost something, I must have been a sight. They informed that someone had turned in a purse at the counter. I enquired about it and yes indeed one good Samaritan saw me leave my purse behind and promptly turned it in. Still to this day I don't know who was so kind to me. I would have loved to have met them and bought them lunch or given them some money. People like that should be rewarded for their acts of kindness. There are more good people out there than we realize.

After surgery, we needed to apply pressure to the area so he wouldn't bleed to death. This was very difficult to do because my father was mean and a bully and would not listen to anybody. He always thought he could do whatever he wanted, rules and good behavior did not apply to him. It made it even harder on me, I explained to the staff what he was like and made excuses. It was one of the most embarrassing times for me. He was abusive to the doctors and nurses and I explained to the staff what he was like. The staff were grateful for the truth because they could get people that were trained to handle this kind of situation. The nurses were changed immediately to accommodate the individual they had before them. My mother did not want anyone knowing what my father was like and became upset with me. I didn't care. I did not want to be in the same room with them. I'd tell him to behave properly because those were the people that poked and prodded you and they wouldn't do it nicely if you were mean to them but he wouldn't listen to me.

He got to go home the same day but my mother refused to look after him and make sure the pressure was applied where they inserted the stents so I stayed most of the day and evening. My housework was piling up and I still made supper for my husband when I got home. At this point in my life I felt overwhelmed.

When I got him home, I had prepared the DNR and Power of Attorney for him to sign. He also said I would be the one to decide what was going to happen to him. In no way was my mother to make any decision with regards to his life.

Templates for these documents are online. Every person should have the following documents completed, with copies in the hands of those who need them, well in advance of an accident or illness. Generic templates are included at the end of this book. You need a DNR, personal directive, and a will or living will.

Here I thought I was going to have a nice life with

my husband, but that was not to be. I still found time for bicycling, which was a very good stress reliever. I found I was exhausted and I couldn't show it because no one cared, nor were they interested in what I was going through.

I had too much weight on my shoulders at this point but I couldn't do anything about it. I would try to take long baths with scented Epsom salts and hoped it would make me relax, if only for a short period of time, I could wash my troubles away.

During that year I made sure I spent a lot of time with my parents. My father could not defend himself and I feared my mother would start to abuse him. This was not beyond the realm of possibilities because they were abusive to me, and to each other, my whole life.

I would not be able to live with myself if this happened, so I made sure nothing out of the ordinary was happening. I asked a lot of questions when I got each of them alone to make sure nothing bad was going on and made sure she was giving him his medications.

I was in charge of their well-being. I was no longer their daughter, now I was the primary caregiver for them both. How I felt was immaterial to them, that was obvious. I was just a tool to be used when it was convenient for them. It wasn't a surprise to me because that's how they had treated me when I was growing up but I still had problems dealing with it. My father's well-being should have been my mother's responsibility but she wanted no part in it. I now saw my father as a frightened little boy who needed looking after.

Emotions of the Year – Working Pages

That year my strongest emotions were: unappreciated, exhausted, withdrawing, wiped, and taken advantage of.

Do you feel unappreciated?

My parents did not care about what this was doing to

me. They didn't see how much time it took to deal with their issues and what it cost me in terms of my life. I was totally unappreciated and used as a tool, at least, that's what it felt like. I told myself I was doing it because I would feel better if I did.

I feel unappreciated because;

_____

Do you feel exhausted?

By the time I got home from helping my parents I was exhausted. I would try to take a bath to relax but found I fell asleep in it, so, I would grab a book and read. I could escape into another world and forget about the day.

I feel exhausted because:

_____

Do you feel like withdrawing?

I began to withdraw from life. I could no longer talk to friends, neighbors, or people of any kind that I met during the days. I lost interest in everything. It was like watching a movie but the problem with that was I was in it, there was no way to avoid it. It took everything in me to start talking to friends or my family about what was happening with my parents, and in the end, it did help.

I feel like withdrawing because:

_____

Do you feel wiped?

I had no energy and just wanted to stay in bed and never get up to face the life I was now beginning with looking after my parents. My mother couldn't care less about what my father was going through and was of no help.

I feel wiped because:

_____

Do you feel like you're being taken advantage of?

They could have done some of the things by themselves but preferred to use my kindness to make me do everything for them and if I didn't, they would make me feel guilty.

I feel like I'm being taken advantage of because:

Tips from the Trenches
(TIP) Find a form of exercise, walking, jogging, or bicycling. It doesn't matter what it is but it will help your stress level go down.

(TIP) Listen to your favorite music or talk show.

(TIP) Read your favorite cartoon or comic strip, online.

What I learned about myself…
Truthfulness helps when dealing with hospitals. They have nurses and doctors that are specifically trained to handle difficult patients. My mother was very angry with me because she didn't want anyone to know what my father was really like. I was able to stand up to her and explain it, before I would cower to them. It was a good change for me. I wasn't afraid of them anymore.

If I was to be responsible for their well-being, I was going to do it my way and that would be better for all of us.

I was able to take charge and not worry about the consequences with my parents. I didn't think it was possible to let go of my past but I could do it now. Everything I had gone through as a child had disappeared. It felt as if it had happened to someone else and not me. I was free of my old life growing up.

On the Lighter Side…
We were bicycling one day and a spoke on the rear tire broke. We were a long way from home at that moment. I had never had that happen to me before. It was

just a matter of time when something would go wrong with a bike and of course it would happen to me. When the spoke broke, it made my rear brake rub on the tire making it much harder to peddle and not to mention the wheel is no longer round.

Going up the hills was quite the challenge for me. I was tired from riding all day and now I worked at it much harder just to get home. I stopped an awful lot and my husband was getting annoyed with me.

I'm trying, I'm trying, but getting annoyed with me wasn't helping. We couldn't swap bikes because he is much taller than me, so, it was up to me to get my stupid bike home. Had my husband or I thought of it at the time, we would have released the back brake and there wouldn't have been a problem. I just wouldn't be able to use my back brake, no big deal, right, well we all use the back brake for the majority. Front brakes could make you fly over the handlebars if you stop too fast. There are hills up and down and going down was very exciting because I didn't want to use my front brake too much and flip over the handlebars. As clumsy as I am it was possible for me to hit the brake and cause myself to fly through the air.

As we are riding along my husband, in his infinite wisdom says to me, "Pedal faster." Don't you think I would pedal faster, if I could? Pedaling faster would not help, I still couldn't get enough momentum going, after all the brake was still on.

12 YEAR FIVE – RECONNOITER

It was apparent that my father would need bypass surgery because the stents did not help. I knew about heart attacks but I didn't expect to have to deal with bypass surgery. Something new on my list of things I didn't know but still it was required of me to deal with it.

I had survived another year as a caregiver for two families. I was still taking my father to his doctor's appointments and was told he would need bypass surgery. It was the most difficult year of all. There was more prep work for me to make sure he was ready for the day of surgery. Pre-op classes, bloodwork, registration, x-rays, and so on.

The day of surgery we were at the hospital by 3:00 a.m. so they could get him prepared for the procedure. I was very nervous and anxious because I did not think my father would make it through the operation. It was going to be a long wait before the surgery was over so I went and found a quiet area to sit down and wait. Meanwhile, my mother said that we should go shopping or do something else. She didn't see any point in waiting and couldn't have cared less about him.

I sat down and waited and she had no choice but to join me. She was very annoyed with me. My father came through surgery but they could not wake him and started asking questions about his health and if he drank. My mother promptly said he does not drink. I told the staff he drank hard alcohol every day. They told me that my father would wake up when he felt like it because alcoholics usually respond in that way, so, for nine days he remained comatose. Had he not woken up at this time they would have to put a tube in him for feeding and would never been able to eat normally. I don't think my father could have handled that because he loved his food.

I drove my mother to the hospital twice a day and

made supper for her because she wouldn't cook for herself. I was at my wits end.

When he woke up after nine days, the hospital called me and told me they had restrained him. That day we went up to visit him and he was strapped down to the bed, yelling and swearing, which he never swore, ever. I was told he punched a nurse and needed to be restrained. Again, I was so embarrassed by his behavior. I did not realize he was having a reaction to one of the medications they gave him, which made him psychotic. They finally changed his medication and he became a bit better. On one visit the staff said he should get up and start walking around the ward. He got his walker and began a trip around the area and looked at my mother and slapped her and pushed her away. The nurses quickly intervened, told my mother to leave and put my father back to his bed and strapped him down. It was so horrible for me. I did not want the staff to know they were my parents. Once again, I told the staff what he was like and they thanked me for the information. The nurses were changed immediately to accommodate my father. People that work in hospitals should be commended for the work they do. I even brought in doughnuts a few times to show them I appreciated their patience with my father.

I was the only one who was allowed to visit with him after that, but my mother would sit in the waiting area to find out how he was doing. Again, my mother should have dealt with this, not me. I wasn't sure why she wanted to come because she didn't really care what happened to him.

After they changed his medication he got back to normal, which isn't saying much, because he was never a nice person. I came in for one visit and saw he was strapped down again. I talked to the nurses and was told he took out his I.V. that he had in his carotid artery. He could have bled to death.

I was so ashamed to call them my family at that

point. On the day we could take my father home, which was a month later, my mother told me I had better stay over. I was not going to do that. It was her responsibility to look after him during the night, not mine. Every morning I stopped by for a visit. When the nurse came by their house to remove my father's stitches, my mother called and said I was to be there. Why me? It was a simple procedure, removing stitches is not a big deal, but she would not let the nurse in if I wasn't there. Talk about parents using their children. I was there for all of it, my mother would not handle anything.

My father was given a lot of medication. He was taking fifteen pills a day, spread out over the course of twenty-four hours. He also slept most of the time, awake for four to five hours. I made sure I went over when he was awake, so I could find out how he was doing, and if he was getting his pills.

I noticed that my mother had a pill box for him that marked the time of day with the pills in it. Most times she didn't pay attention and he would get two pills that were the same and miss others. I would sort them out properly and check the next day if he got them. Sadly, no, she mixed them up again. When my father got up, he immediately went and took the pills again.

My father was on insulin and he gave himself the shot when he got up in the morning and when I arrived, he would take the insulin again. This would put him into another coma because he was taking double the dose. Back to the hospital we went. He spent half his time in the hospital over the course of the year which meant I was taking my mother to the hospital every day.

At one point the staff talked to me and were worried for his well-being. I was asked if he was getting his pills and I had no choice but to say that he was taking them two at a time, getting his insulin more often than he should or missing them entirely, and my mother was mixing up his medications. I was worried for him too but there was nothing I could do at the time, even when I explained it to my mother, she said she didn't care about any of it. It wasn't her problem.

One time while visiting my parents I asked where my father was and she responded with, 'I don't know.' I started searching for him inside and outside of the house and he was nowhere. I began to panic. Surely, he couldn't have gone far because he refused to walk after his bypass because it hurt too much. An hour had elapsed when I heard a noise in the basement. I went down to look and sure enough there was my father crawling around under the basement stairs. He said he was looking for something and it took a few minutes but I did manage to convince him to come back upstairs.

That year was a complete fiasco for me and I was at a loss of what to do. Everything I did my mother would undermine me. I told her no more painkillers but she gave them to my father anyway. I made sure his pills were put in his pill box correctly and when I left, she would mix them up again. It was an issue I had no control over and it concerned me. I would not be able to live with the guilt if something happened to my father while in the care of my mother so I spent even more time at their house. I worried every night about him and if he was okay.

Emotions of the Year – Working Pages

That year the strongest emotions I had were: a nightmare, despair, hell, screaming, hit something.

Do you feel your life is a nightmare?

I was positive my life was now a nightmare. I was at my wits end. I didn't know what to do or who I could turn to. Everyone around me was sick. I saw no way out. I started to remember I felt like that when my husband got sick and reminded myself, every day, that it would get better.

I feel my life is a nightmare because:

_____

Do you feel despair?

I was missing out on life, the beauty around me, and I couldn't see anything good about my life. I would walk around the hospital while I waited for my father to go through his procedures. I noticed there were other people doing the same thing as me. I was glad to see I wasn't the only one going through this. Talking to others at the hospital made me realize the illness may not be the same but the caregiving was. Had I have gone to a support group I would have seen others and how they dealt with the situation. But sadly, I did not.

I feel despair because:

_____

Do you feel like you're living in hell?

Never a kind word was said to me by my parents. They were both selfish and self-serving. It was up to me to pat myself on the back and say encouraging words that would help me get through this. I took on the job as a caregiver for my parents because they would not know what to do and were helpless and I was duty bound to make sure they received the best care. I didn't do it to get praise, I did it because I loved them, but sometimes a nice word would have been appreciated.

I feel like I'm living in hell because:

_____

Do you just want to scream?

I could not believe that this was my life. I wanted to scream. Everything became surreal. I lost myself and I missed who I was becoming after my husband's recovery, even if it was for a short period of time. I needed to make the time for me and so I did. Hot baths always work.

I want to scream because:

_____

Do you want to hit something?

There were days I just wanted to hit something, anything. I took that anger and went for a walk and while walking I would start crying. I always found crying to help.

I feel like I want to hit something because:

_____

Tips from the Trenches

(TIP) Reach out to someone, talk to a nurse or a family doctor, they may have a useful suggestion to help you through it.

(TIP) Cook big meals, and share between households. Do batch cooking and store portions in the freezer for easy suppers on harder days.

(TIP) Try something new. Your focus will be on the new idea rather than what you are going through.

What I learned about myself…

I couldn't control everything around me. I had to learn how to trust other people and hope they would do the right thing. I would help when I was needed and not try to be in charge all of the time. It was hard at first but it became easier as the days passed by.

I started to research the medications and why they were prescribed and by doing so I learned some were not required. It was like learning a new language. I became knowledgeable on the medical side of things and was proud of myself for doing it. I wanted to be the best I could be in regards to caregiving for my loved ones and I was.

On the Lighter Side…

One day we were out pedaling our bikes and for some reason my husband says to me, "let's reconnoiter at the corner". Sure, I can do that if only I knew what that meant at the time.

I started heading for home and suddenly my husband was no longer with me. I guess he wanted to go at his own speed and we would meet at home later. Off I went. It was late at night and no moon out. I decided it would be better if I walked the bike home. While doing this I kept my bike on my right which was closest to the edge of the curb. I tripped on the sidewalk and fell onto the road on top of my bike. When I got home, my husband wasn't there. I looked in a mirror and saw I had a huge lump on my forehead and a bruise was emerging. I think at that point I was suffering a concussion. I had all the symptoms and my husband still wasn't home. After an hour he finally shows up and he's upset.

I say, "what's up, what happened to you?" He responded with, "I told you to reconnoiter at the corner.

If I knew what the word meant at the time, I would have complied but as it was, it was the first time I ever heard that word. I looked it up and all it means is to meet up at some place. Couldn't he have just said to meet him at the corner?

I did consider bringing along a dictionary on future rides, that way there would be no confusion when he wanted to use words I didn't know. How stupid would I look if I brought a dictionary with me on my bike and pulled it out whenever he used words I didn't know? Never mind that I was experiencing a concussion and he never asked how I got a big lump on my head. Really?

13 YEAR SIX – I CAN'T SEE YOU

I had made it through another year only to find myself totally overwhelmed by my responsibilities. Looking after elderly people is very hard. They are stubborn and think they know everything. I started taking another university course, thinking it might help because I was doing something for me, but they took up so much time that I quit.

Running between my house and my parents' house was awful. I had no time to do anything else. My mother hated my father because she was jealous, I spent so much time helping my father and not spending time with her. I would have preferred it if she looked after him, but she, instead, resented him. I had to stop them from fighting with each other and I remember there was an incident, when I called emergency. When I arrived, my parents had something in their hands and I believed at that time they would have hurt each other with it. My mother was screaming when I got there and she was telling him to move out. I could not get them to tell me what happened, they were yelling at the top of their lungs at each other. I called 911, I needed help. When the emergency responders arrived, (fire truck, police, and ambulance), my mother was yelling and telling everyone to get him out of her house. I was questioned about the situation but I couldn't help them, I had no answers. They took my father down to the basement and I was supposed to get my mother calm. That was much easier said than done. I realized in this situation I had no choice but to call in help, even my life was in danger, it took most of the day to get the crisis under control and eventually they relinquished their weapons and we got them calmed down enough that we could all leave. It truly was a frightening day. There are times when you cannot help and have to seek outside assistance. I had no choice but to do what I did even when my mother was mad at me for calling strangers to help me in this situation.

Life!!! What does one do in this situation? My mother hated my father and my father was sick. So, now I was spending even more time at their house and try to keep the peace.

There was way too much drama in my life and all the while I still looked after my husband.

I got so good at finding my way around hospitals, that I actually helped people who were lost and didn't know where to go, to get to the room they needed to be at. They were always grateful and asked if I worked at the hospital. I would just tell them that I spent way too much time in hospitals and leave it at that. I felt really good when I helped perfect strangers out who were scared and didn't know who to ask for directions. Hospitals are scary places to be and I understood that.

My life was hell! I was still able to help my husband, look after the house, cook, etc. Some days I just felt like pulling the covers over my head to make the world go away but that was not my lot in life. So onwards and upwards I went to face another day. I truly hated my life, it wasn't easy, and it wasn't fair. I knew deep down inside no one was to blame and I did not want my father to be abused or suffer more than he already was. It was difficult for him because he was always a strong independent man before he got sick and now, he was fragile.

Looking after my husband after his heart attack was hard in the beginning but I soon started to enjoy doing it, he was so different from my father. My husband would try to do things for himself and my father did nothing that would help him get better. My mother should have been the one doing the lion's share of the work, not me.

I was so angry, frustrated, and depressed. I did what was required of me and nobody saw what I was going through because I didn't let it show. I took long walks in the evening so I might feel better, and sometimes it helped, other times a long hot bath would do it.

My father required many doctor visits. He now had four doctors, each dealing with a different issue. He had nerve damage and was in a lot of pain. The pills he was given said no alcohol, but my mother would always give him some, so the pills did nothing for him. I would explain to the doctor what was happening and he just said that was up to them. If they didn't want to follow the advice it was on them.

My mother would not take my father to the doctors' appointments or fill his prescriptions so I did it. I had no choice. I would not see my father suffer because my mother wouldn't step up, that wasn't right. Again, I would not have been able to live with myself knowing I could have done something to help my father. My mother had already proven she was incapable of looking after him.

I was still making the doctors' appointments for my husband too. I would sit on hold for hours at a time trying to get hold of doctors' offices and found it very frustrating and there was nothing I could do about it, I felt helpless.

This aspect of my life was just so horrible. Explaining to doctors what was happening to my father was very difficult. My parents just didn't listen to me. I could not abandon them, I felt sorry for my father. My parents were never kind, just the opposite. They were both abusive towards me while I was growing up but they told me at a young age that when they got old, I would have to look after them and so I did and still do today. I have always done what is expected of me, even to this day. They told me that they would never go to a retirement home or nursing home. That was why they had me.

I always felt under-appreciated, used, and taken advantage of. It isn't nice to think of your parents that way, but I did. They didn't even try to do things for themselves.

I was ashamed of them most times and at some

point, I didn't know if I should help them or just leave them to do whatever they wanted but I wouldn't be able to live with myself if I walked away.

I distanced my feelings as their daughter and treated it as I was their caregiver, that way I would not be embarrassed by their behavior. It made quite a difference to me thinking in those terms, not a daughter but a caregiver.

Emotions of the Year – Working Pages

That year the strongest emotions I had were: out of control, depressed, confused, impatient, overwhelmed.

Do you feel out of control?

I felt my life was out of control, I wasn't able to do the things that made me feel better about myself, which in turn, would make me a better caregiver. I started taking one of my hobbies with me that I liked to do, over to my parents' house or hospital. When they talked, I responded, but I really wasn't paying too much attention.

I feel out of control because:

_____

Do you feel depressed?

I found that there was a dark cloud over me. I was depressed and did not want to be alive anymore. This was a very dark period for me and I needed to figure out some way that I could overcome it. I decided to take up jogging and it did help. It was hard to find the time but I managed to fit it in.

I feel depressed because:

_____

Do you feel confused?

I was running on fumes and wasn't sure which way to turn so I sat down and started writing. Everything I felt was written down on paper. I realized that I could now compartmentalize my life. I had a life as a wife to my husband and a daughter to my parents, I separated the two and dealt with it accordingly.

I feel confused because:

_____

Do you feel impatient?

I lacked patience when it came to my parents. They would not listen or understand what they were doing to me, so I would go home and talk to my husband or girlfriend about how I felt. Talking to someone helps a lot.

I feel impatient because:

_____

Do you feel overwhelmed?

Feeling overwhelmed was taking up too much time, it exhausted me. I still helped my husband with his issues and still found time to bicycle with him during the summer. Spending time with someone else made all the difference to me. I was having fun with him and it didn't feel like a chore.

I feel overwhelmed because:

_____

Tips from the Trenches

(TIP) There will be situations that arise and sometimes you will need outside help. Don't be afraid to ask for it.

(TIP) Emergency responders are trained to handle difficult situations that you have never faced before. If you or your loved ones are in immediate danger, call your local emergency number. Do not try to handle the situation yourself.

(TIP) Use the hotlines in your area. You can find the number online. Where I live it's 811.

What I learned about myself…

I cared about my parents more than I thought I

did. I would have felt guilty if I did not help them. It may have been overwhelming most days but I felt better about myself for helping them. I wanted to help, that surprised me. I found I loved them more than I thought I did.

I began to learn to have more patience with them, it was also scary for them, and I hadn't realized it. I thought that I was being used and instead it was because they were frightened. They didn't know how to handle the crises before them. On the good days, I noticed the life around me. People were kind, birds were singing, and life was happening all around me every day. I felt better seeing the nice things about life. It became a coping mechanism for me.

On the Lighter Side…

I had Saturday's off as a caregiver. I would ride with my husband through the parks. We would stop at a convenience store and get crackers, tomatoes, cheese, and sausage. When we arrived at the park we would sit and enjoy having a picnic.

I was getting good at riding up the hills and some hills were quite steep but my husband was faster getting up them then I was. When the path was relatively flat, I gained speed and got quite far ahead.

There were park benches along the way that I never stopped at. I did not know my husband wanted me to stop at them, so I asked him, "Why didn't you tell me to stop." He always responded with, "I can't see you, how am I supposed to tell you to stop?" Oh, right! He told me every time he saw a bench, he hoped I would be sitting on it waiting for him to catch up with me but I kept on going. I was on a mission to get to the final park and eat my greasy burger. That was our reward for riding through the park systems in the city and it was always the best burger we could have because you build up quite an appetite while riding.

I get it. I was too far ahead. We bought walkie-talkies after that. Thinking about it later it wasn't such a good idea because when you're flying down a hill one cannot or must not use the walkie-talkie. Do not take your hands off of the handlebars. I remember a phrase from when I was a kid, "Look mom, no hands, look mom no feet, look mom no teeth," and that wouldn't turn out well. Still, to this day we have never used them and probably never will.

14 YEAR SEVEN – MY DAUGHTER TAKES A TIME-OUT, NOT THE DOG

By the time the seventh year of me being a caregiver arrived, I was getting everything under control. I managed my life and my parents' life quite well. I even found time to do things I enjoyed and I could see life getting better.

It had now become much simpler. I only visited my parents once a week. It was nice, I had more free time to explore who I was and who I wanted to become. I still spent a lot of time with my husband and I never felt like I was a caregiver to him anymore. He was a survivor and a fighter.

We found that we spent a lot of time just sitting together and talking for hours on end. We had made it. Life was amazing.

The year had many opportunities for me and I took them. It was a year of me being proud of myself, I was confident, I could be whatever I wanted to be because of what I did for everyone else. I became strong and could handle anything.

My husband was no longer depressed or angry. He was happy again and it was nice to see.

We got a rescued puppy and the moment I saw her she was mine. She was full of life and crazy. She was happy to have a home and we were ecstatic to have her. I got to spend all my time with her and it was wonderful to have a dog again.

She became my dog. She went everywhere with me. We were inseparable and still are today.

My daughter always tells me raising a child or puppy is also being a caregiver but I have never felt that. Watching someone grow up and seeing the wonder in their eyes when they discover something new does not feel like

I am being a caregiver. I still don't see it as being a caregiver, today.

When I didn't know what to do with myself, I would get my dog and we would go for a long walk. I saw the splendor in the world. I was happy to be alive. My dog was so thrilled to be alive and having a home and a family that we got energy just by being around her.

She hated it when my husband went to work. We had a mirror on the headboard of our bed and she would run in and look at the mirror and howl, run back out and do it in front of my husband, making a sad face. You could practically hear her thoughts, "if I just look sad enough, dad will stay home". She would do it two or three times before my husband left but it never worked. He always went out the door. Other times she would sit and practice her saddest faces in front of the mirror so she would be prepared the next day.

One time my husband took our dog for a walk and it was hot out. He wanted to get her some water and found a fast food outlet. Can't bring the dog inside so he went through the drive-through. When he got to the window the lady said he was not allowed to do that. I'm not sure why you can't, it makes no sense, but I still laugh to this day picturing my husband moving in the line of cars to get our dog some water. What must the people be thinking in their vehicles?

I was happy again and enjoying my life. When I went on a job for our business, I took my dog. Our clients didn't mind if I brought her in with me. They all seemed to be dog people. That was nice.

I worked when there was work for me and everything was going great. My husband was doing very well and my parents did not need me anymore, all the time. I would visit my parents when I wanted to and not because they needed me.

I found it to be an amazing year. I was busy but it was all about me doing the things I liked and discovered other things I wanted to do. I could conquer anything and I felt good about myself.

I tackled all my hobbies and enjoyed myself. That year was such a fantastic year for me. I had my whole life to look forward to. It was all about me and I was loving every moment of it.

I'm glad I didn't waste a minute of it because I thought my life as a caregiver was over but it didn't work out that way. At least I had almost a year off and I got to recharge my batteries.

Emotions of the Year – Working Pages

That year the strongest emotions I had were: relieved, satisfied, proud, impressed, joy.

Do you feel relieved?

It was seven years of caregiving and I was tired but I felt relief because this year looked much better for me. I spent less time with my parents and more time with my husband.

I feel relieved because:

_____

Do you feel satisfied?

I was satisfied with everything I had done. I couldn't think of anything I could have done better for everyone, so I sometimes took myself shopping and buy something nice just for me.

I feel satisfied because:

_____

Do you feel proud?

I found I felt proud of what I had done and accomplished as a caregiver, and that was a nice feeling for me.

I feel proud because:

_____

Do you feel impressed by what you did?

Seven years had passed by and I realized I had become an amazing person. I never knew I had it in me until I went through it.

I feel impressed by what I did because:

_____

Do you feel joy?

I was once again smiling and laughing. I saw the beauty around me. My life was once again mine and things were looking up.

I feel joy because:

_____

Tips from the Trenches

(TIP) Enjoy the down-time because you don't know how long it will last. Don't' waste a moment, embrace it. Do something that you enjoy whenever possible. You never know when the next crisis will occur.

(TIP) Squeeze a stress ball. You can find one anywhere, even the dollar store. I wore mine out.

(TIP) Petting an animal or playing with one lightens your mood.

What I learned about myself…

I enjoyed being by myself. I had never liked being alone but now I did. My dog had so much energy that it was hard to not to be infected by it. I was on top of the world. I discovered I wanted to learn to cook gourmet dishes and I already had the cook books to do so.

I was taking my dog for walks during the day and enjoying it, that was something I never would have done before. I was still changing and growing each and every day for the better. I would stop and chit chat with strangers while walking my dog and they theirs. We exchanged funny stories about our dogs and would continue laughing as we parted ways.

On the Lighter Side…

My daughter was living in another city and she would come see us when she could. I told her we had a new rescued puppy and sent her pictures. On one visit she met the new addition to our family. This dog was over the moon to find out she even got a kid in the deal.

It didn't matter that my daughter was in her thirties at the time, the dog was ecstatic. The dog was all over her all the time.

One morning my daughter wanted to sleep in and my dog had other ideas. She put the covers over her head to get away from the dog but the dog was having none of it. The dog poked her head under the blankets anyway. She annoyed my daughter so much that when I got up, I looked outside and my daughter was standing outside in her pajama's.

"Why are you standing outside in the cold?", I asked.

"I need a time-out your dog is crazy."

I get it. She's a loony dog but she was just so happy to see my daughter first thing in the morning. I think my dog should have had a time-out and not the other way around but there it is. My daughter gave herself a time-out instead and over the next year the dog calmed down and my daughter was able to sleep in.

15 YEAR EIGHT - MY DOG HAS AN IDEA

Everything was going along great and then one day, our friends came to visit, and mentioned that Hubbie did not look well. I didn't see the change in my husband but they were right when I stopped and looked at him. His skin became ashy in color and he didn't have any energy. I asked him about how he was feeling but his response was his usual, "I feel fine".

My husband had a yearly appointment with his cardiologist so we waited until we could talk to him. We could not call in to make an earlier appointment for him. Waiting is the hardest part.

He told me when he took a breath, his lungs felt like they were burning. I had no words for him. I didn't know what was happening to him this time. I was scared, I didn't know what to do.

Every time our friends saw him, they reminded me that he did not look well. I didn't want to hear that. What was I supposed to do?

The day arrived and the doctor said he would need stents. His arteries were clogged. The waiting list was long and we wouldn't get in until the following year for his procedure. At least this time I knew what to expect. It was only going to take a morning and he would begin to feel better right away.

No more walking or bicycling for him. He was to take it easy and not do anything stressful until after the procedure. It was hard to make him do nothing, he was always very active. He got angry, scared, and depressed again, and so did I.

I was terrified of losing my husband once again. It was difficult to see him that way. He never knew how I felt and he never should. I could see him getting weaker and sicker each day. I hoped that we could get the procedure done faster but that was not the case.

I helped as much as I could with our business that year, making it less stressful for him, or so I hoped. It did help but the work load became great for me. I was doing it all again. I was slowly going into a depression again. I saw no hope with life or me. The dark cloud appeared once again in our lives.

I could not believe that all life had in store for me was me being a caregiver for the rest of my life. I wanted more but could not have it. I was crying for me this time because I could not do the things I wanted and I was angry at my husband for putting me through all this again.

I knew it wasn't his fault but I didn't care. It was because of him I was dealing with his health issues again. I went from having such a good and wonderful year to this. A life of fear!

We were both angry but for different reasons. I was mad at him for getting sick again and he was mad at himself. I felt so guilty for feeling like that but that was what I felt and nobody could take that away from me.

I hid my feelings from everyone, I kept them inside. I wasn't able to go for walks because that would make my husband feel bad and besides, he would have wanted to go with me. This did not help the situation at all. Neither of us got any exercise for the rest of the year.

It was hard for my husband being stagnant for eight months, I could see it but there was nothing either of us could do about the situation, we just needed to wait and waiting is the hardest part.

Emotions of the Year – Working Pages

That year the strongest emotions I had were: bad, worthless, sick, tired, and fed up.

Do you feel bad?

I totally missed the signs that there was something

wrong with my husband and I felt horrible. He sometimes complained when he took a breath that his lungs burned. He refused to see the doctor. I did understand he was fed up with doctors and everything that entailed, so we ignored it. That was not the right thing to do.

I feel bad because:

_____

Do you feel worthless?

How horrible can a person feel when you miss all the signs of someone getting sick? I was very upset with myself but I couldn't do anything about it so I tried reading or doing a crossword puzzle.

I feel worthless because:

_____

Do you feel sick?

I started getting sick, I would get heart palpitations, and I began throwing up just from the stress alone. I didn't want to have to go through it again. Our family doctor reassured me that nothing was wrong with me.

I feel sick because:

_____

Do you feel tired?

I found I had no energy and was always tired. It was hard to get up some mornings. I still embraced the day and carried on. I even went to the extent of getting plug-in fragrances that would help me feel better.

I feel tired because:

_____

Do you feel fed up?

I felt like giving up, how much can one person endure? It was back to the same feelings I had before and there was nothing I could do about it. I made sure that each day I did one thing for myself, whatever I thought would cheer me up. I did not want to lose myself this time.

I feel fed up because:

_____

Tips from the Trenches

(TIP) Don't forget to look after yourself. You're just as important as your loved one and you can't care for someone else if you get sick. Take care yourself, you'll be able to cope with the situation better.

(TIP) Get a Power of Attorney in place. The hospital may have some or else there are free ones online.

(TIP) Find out if you need a 'DO NOT RESUCITATE' (DNR), if that is what your loved one wants done.

What I learned about myself...

I needed to look after myself. At first, I felt guilty about doing it but after a while, I realized I could handle situations much better if I did it. it became a necessity rather than a luxury. There were still many bad days but self-care was important and it made me cope better with the situation.

I learned better ways to handle the stress so it wouldn't overwhelm me again. I took the time to read, sew, or draw. I made the time. I took the time. I had no choice because otherwise I would be getting sick to the point that I would need a caregiver and then who would look after my family?

On the Lighter Side...

Our dog was still as crazy as ever. I don't know where she found it but she found a light bulb in our yard. Someone must have thrown it over the fence which begs the question 'why would you carry a light bulb outside and throw it into your neighbor's yard. I have always kept a clean yard and garden and I never noticed the bulb being there.

I let our dog in and what did I see but our dog holding the light bulb in her mouth with the glass part inside. I panicked and called for my husband. I didn't want her to bite down on it and she would listen to him more than she listened to me.

My husband removed the light bulb without an incident. He looked at me, "I think our dog has an idea". Yeah, not funny but it made me think of the cartoons when they draw a light bulb over their heads indicating that they thought of something.

My husband may have been sick but he could still pull off the one-liners and still to this day he has that ability.

16 YEAR NINE – OH, LOOK, IT'S A CANOE, OH, LOOK, IT'S A FLOAT

April finally came and we had done all the pre-op procedures. We now had a date for the stents. I was glad to see the day come so that my husband would once again feel better. Receiving stents is no big deal, they let you go home the same day, so I was looking forward to it.

First off, in this country we cannot sue the medical profession or pharmaceutical companies.

The doctors put too many stents in and one of them blew up very close to his heart and caused his heart to stop, they revived him, and he suffered another heart attack.

I was sitting in the room waiting for half an hour after they took him in for the procedure when the next thing I know, the doctor comes to me and says your husband just suffered another heart attack.

I started shaking and crying. I was by myself. They asked if they could contact someone for me, I said no, I asked how long it would be before I could see my husband, and the doctor said he didn't even know if my husband was going to make it, that was the most horrible thing to hear.

I went out to the sitting area and texted our daughter about what had just happened to her dad. At that time, she lived six hours away and it was a long drive for her. She packed up her cat and sundry items and drove to the hospital as quick as she could. By the time she got to me, I still had not been able to see my husband. Nobody came and told me what was going on.

What a sight my daughter and I were, we just sat there crying, we didn't care if anyone saw us. They finally came and told us later that evening that we would not be able to see my husband until the next day.

We went to the hospital first thing the next morning and found my husband strapped down and yelling. Because of what my father went through being psychotic from the medication, I was well aware of what was happening to my husband. My daughter was scared to death but I reassured her he would be fine, I just needed to talk to the nurse and tell her he was reacting badly to that medication. It took four days for him to recover from the reaction and still to this day he remembers nothing of it.

During that time the nurses would tell me I couldn't go into the room because of whatever they were doing and the next thing I knew he was yelling my name and the nurses would let me in. At least he never forgot my name or who I was during that time.

He remained in the hospital for ten days and one of the doctors' told us the truth about why the procedure didn't work. Only one doctor admitted the truth and the next day promptly denied what he said. It never happened.

While my husband remained in the hospital the doctor told us he would need a pacemaker and they would be doing the procedure the next morning. He did not get breakfast and by the time I got there he told me they did not give him a pacemaker. He wasn't allowed a meal before the procedure but he also didn't get lunch after. This happened over and over for the next ten days. Nothing to eat before and they just forgot about him after they cancelled the procedure. I was not amused. I watched my husband losing the will to live more each day.

One time a nurse came in and said they were going to weigh him. He weighed 195 pounds when I brought him in and when he stepped on the scale the nurse said he weighed 220 lbs. My husband promptly told the nurse the scale is broken, he did not weigh that much. He is the only person I know that can gain weight on hospital food. The food in hospitals is horrible.

Next time I came in I brought a tomato with me and my husband says I don't know what I would give to have a tomato right now. Well, I just happened to bring one and gave it to him. Next thing he says, it would taste much better if I had some salt. Hmmm, I just happen to have some with me. It was the best tomato he had ever had, that day.

I had enough with the staff jerking us around and finally said I wanted to speak to the doctor because I was taking him home. As soon as my husband found out he was going to be able to go home his spirits got much better. The doctor advised us it was a bad decision. I said I didn't care because they weren't doing anything. I signed a paper saying I was responsible for anything that went wrong with him by taking him home. That to me was not a problem. I would bring him in on the day they would actually do the procedure but they never called. He did not require a pacemaker so I don't know what that was all about. I wish the doctor would have explained why they wanted the procedure done and why they didn't do it because I needed to make sense of it.

Now, I was back on the job looking after Hubbie. At this point, I was fed up with my job as a caregiver. This didn't seem fair to me. No one saw it, but I was very angry that I would have to do this forever. There was no end in sight and I dealt with this on my own.

This time, though, I knew what all the stages of recovery were, and started from scratch with Hubbie, so he would recover fully. At least, I knew what I was doing this time.

It was hard for my husband because once again, it wasn't his fault, and we needed to deal with all of it. How many times does a person have to go through another crisis before it stops?

This time it was taking much longer because my husband did not want to go through the road of recovery again. He had given up. His ability to read vanished again and he would have to start over training his brain to focus and retain what he was reading. I felt bad for him.

Watching him go through it again and not being able to help with his reading was hard to see.

I was now working full time again with our business and looking after him. It was a very dark period for the both of us. This was not supposed to be happening again. I dealt with everything, work, home, friends, and family. Not what I had envisioned my life would be and there it was anyway.

My daughter was trying her hardest to move back to her home town so she could be near her Dad. She gave up her career and was starting again back home.

I was glad to know she was coming home because seeing her on the weekends always made me feel better. We always had fun together, no matter what. We always laughed and joked around. She is my best friend and I love her dearly.

The hospital wanted to remedy their mistake and booked him in for triple bypass surgery eight months later which would be in the following year.

Emotions of the Year – Working Pages

That year the strongest emotions I had were: running away, breaking something, pity, resentment, detached.

Do you feel like running away?

I felt like running away. The burden was too great for me to handle. I made myself stop feeling anything anymore, it just wasn't worth it. I became numb.

I feel like running away because:

_____

Do you want to break something?

I wanted to break things, throw things, punch a wall, but I didn't. Oh, but I so wanted to. I don't think it would have made me feel better but there it was.

I feel like breaking something because:

_____

Do you feel pity?

I felt sorry for myself, not my husband. It was too much for me. This year became a nightmare and I felt pity for myself.

I feel pity because:

_____

Do you feel resentment?

I hated life and I hated my husband for everything he put me through. I dug deep within myself to find the love I felt for him and the empathy I had because it truly wasn't his fault, not this time.

I feel resentment because:

_____

Do you feel detached?

It felt like I was looking down on someone else's life. This could not be happening again. I had a feeling of detachment, I was numb, I wasn't feeling anything anymore.

I feel detached because:

_____

Tips from the Trenches

(TIP) Find some humor in every situation you encounter. Laughter is still the best medicine.

(TIP) Make sure your loved one has a will or a living will in place.

(TIP) Check out monthly parking passes if it's going to be an extended time in the hospital.

What I learned about myself…

Doctors and nurses are not infallible. I saw what was happening to my husband while he stayed in the hospital and I took charge. I had the courage to stand up to the doctor and explain the situation to him. My husband was getting worse and they weren't dealing with the problem. I understand the doctors and nurses are very busy and cannot treat each patient differently, but I was going to lose my husband if he was not released. I had the strength to take matters into my own hands. I had never done that before. I was still changing. In the end, I was right because my husband didn't require a pacemaker.

On the Lighter Side…

My daughter was moving back to her home town. We were both very excited to have her near us again. On one drive to the hospital she and I were waiting at the traffic lights and we saw a canoe drive past us in the crosswalk in front of her car. We were both tired and didn't know what to say about it, were we hallucinating or just imagining it. Neither of us wanted to say, "did you see that?" But no, it was a recumbent bike made to look like a canoe, you couldn't see his pedals or handlebars, he did a really good job of disguising his bike. When he went by us and was gone, we both admitted to seeing a canoe float past us.

When we were leaving the hospital, my daughter said she wanted to live in this area. It is a nice area but as we were driving, all I could do is point my finger so she would look at what I was seeing.

Use your words she said to me. No way, first it was a canoe and now I was seeing another bicycle except this one had so many bells and whistles on it, it looked like it should be in a parade.

My daughter started laughing and exclaimed, "Oh, look, it's a float." That's what it looked like, a float that belongs in a parade. Needless to say, after that day my daughter decided to look for an apartment in another part of the city. I was glad, that neighborhood was weird.

I told my husband about this float and he said yup this guy decorates his bike for every special day of the year. I don't know how he pedal with all that weight on his bicycle but he did and my husband saw the guy all the time when he drove through the area.

17 YEAR TEN – A BANDAGE HOLDING STITCHES TOGETHER

By the time February came we were glad that he would be having bypass surgery because the stents did not work, that was obvious. It had all gone horribly wrong the previous year.

In 2011 my husband went through triple bypass surgery. I had already been through it with my father and knew what to expect, or so I thought. I went through all the same emotions as I did with my father but they were two different people and came through the surgery differently.

The surgery took longer than expected and so I became scared and I was crying, not again, I thought, something must have gone wrong. It took longer because at the time, I did not know, we had gotten the best heart surgeon in the hospital. By the time the doctor came and told us he was ok and doing very well, my daughter and I, were both a wreck. It had been a very long day for us.

By the time we got to the hospital, the next day, my husband was doing laps around the ward. I knew he must be in a lot of pain but he didn't show it. He wanted to go home as soon as possible. He had gone in on Thursday and doing laps Friday morning. His surgeon, which surprised everyone, came in on Sunday to see how he was doing and next thing we knew he was coming the doctor said he could go home the next day.

My husband was and is a fighter. He was so happy to find out that he would be coming home so soon. He still had a tube in him that could not be removed for a few days but nobody cared. His place was at home where I could look after him once again.

They cracked his ribs open and took out veins from his leg so, he didn't have much mobility. He hated having to rely on me for the simple things a person takes for granted. I would help him put on his socks and shoes. I didn't mind, he was still alive, and that was all that mattered to me.

It was hard for him to get into a vehicle and out. The roads were too bumpy, everything hurt for him and I couldn't fix it. I was now responsible for taking him to his surgeon, his cardiologist, and our family doctor, many times during that year.

It didn't take long until he tried to do everything on his own but you could see he was mad, angry, frustrated, and fed up with everything he was going through. "Well, what about me?", I thought. I was the caregiver and I wasn't happy either and couldn't show it. Again, I was feeling sorry for myself and not looking at my life like I should. It would get better, it did before. I just couldn't see it at the time.

I went through the motions every day, I got up, helped Hubbie, went to work, came home, did all the stuff required at home, and went to bed. This time, though, it only took a year for Hubbie to get better.

He was feeling better every day and progress was being made on his part. I, on the other hand, was exhausted. How much stress can the human body go through before it just stops?

I was completely numb by the end of the year it had become too much for me to deal with. Between my husband and my father, which I was glad they managed to get sick separately and not together, I was at a stage in my life where running away was my only solution. I didn't, but I really wanted to. I wanted to walk out the front door and never come back.

I was glad my husband was doing so well but I just wanted the world to end for me. I did not think I had anything left to give at the time but looking back that was not the worst year, it was to come a few years later.

95

Emotions of the Year – Working Pages

That year the strongest emotions I had were: stunned, inadequate, unimportant, distant, and nothing.

Do you feel stunned?

It felt like someone had hit me in the head with a 2x4. I did not know what to feel at this point. I was overwhelmed and could not feel much of anything at the time.

I feel stunned because:

_____

Do you feel inadequate?

I did not feel like I was doing anything right anymore. I went through the motions but I didn't think I was useful, inadequate, comes to mind but I struggled through.

I feel inadequate because:

_____

Do you feel unimportant?

My life didn't matter, it was all about my husband and what he was going through, even with friends and family. I wasn't important to anybody, what I was going through, nobody cared.

I feel unimportant because:

_____

Do you feel distant?

I became very distant. No one wanted to hear about me, only what my husband was going through and feeling. It just didn't seem right to me so I withdrew.

I feel distant because:

_____

Do you feel anything?

I once again started feeling numb and unappreciated. I shut down completely. I felt nothing, nothing at all and I was not about to start again.

I don't feel anything because:

_____

Tips from the Trenches
(TIP) Don't go it alone. Use the resources available to you.

(TIP) There are live chat lines online if you need to talk to someone anytime, day or night.

(TIP) Meditate if you can or do some yoga.

What I learned about myself…

I was the only one responsible for my well-being and happiness. I could not enjoy life if I continued to feel sorry for myself or have bouts of depression. I began to take one day at a time and start healing once again and by doing so, I started feeling better. I was able to stop and assess the situation and deal with it and fix it. I worked at feeling good about myself and the way I was handling everything.

On the Lighter Side…

My husband's stitches went all the way down his ribcage. They were healing well. It was now summer and a few months had passed. It was hot out and he took his shirt off. Still to this day you can see where the stitches are.

He put one small bandage on the bottom of his ribs because it bled where he scratched it. The stitches were itchy while they were healing up and in his infinite wisdom, he scratched one too many times.

Our friends came over one day and were staring at my husband and laughing. They looked at him and said, "Do you really think that one little bandage is going to help?"

It really looked strange having one little bandage on when his scar was 8 inches long.

18 YEAR ELEVEN – LASSIE, IS TIMMY IN THE WELL?

By 2012, Hubbie was able to work on his own, so that was good. He was doing amazingly well for what he had gone through. At this point, I thought that I would get some me time but that was not the case.

It was the start of the new-year and all was going well. My father started complaining that he didn't feel well at all and I could see he was beginning to deteriorate. I talked to my husband about what was happening with my father and would it be alright if we bought a bigger house and they would be able to move in with us. At this point, I need to tell you that they had lived with us before for eight years. They never really did well on their own together. My mother and father never liked living alone, they always wanted me to look after them, even when they weren't sick, so this was not out of the norm.

I brought the idea up with my parents and they jumped at the chance, but only if I got to pick the area where I would live. I had always wanted to live in the country all my life, so this was my opportunity, and I went forward with it.

Now came the problem, I sold both of our houses and found a new home that my mother and I would like. It was March when I put the houses up for sale and two weeks later, I had once again placed my father in the hospital. I didn't know what was happening with him health wise but needless to say, I did it all. My father's signature was required for the sale of their house. This was going to be difficult because the lawyers needed to know if he was lucid and knew what was going on with this matter. He passed the test and everything moved forward.

I was visiting my father twice a day and at the same time preparing for the move. I had found a home that my mother and I both agreed on and signed the deal.

The hospital said that my father would not be able to live with my mother alone anymore. She was not strong enough to help him if he fell down and so they would be placing him in a nursing home when one became available. The wait was going to be two years. I would be visiting him in the hospital for the duration.

I dealt with everything on my own. Lawyer's appointments, packing up both houses, arranging the dates for the sale of both houses and the day of the move. My girlfriend was amazing, every day she would call me and find out which house we would be packing on that day. She was with me every day helping me pack. My mother was useless and did not know what to do, all she was required to do was start packing, but she couldn't even do that and all the while I was still driving my mother to the hospital twice a day and making supper for her and us.

I don't know where I got the energy to accomplish everything but somehow, I managed and I did it very well. It was one of the most organized moves I have ever seen and our new neighbors said they were impressed at how well I did with the move. Moving trucks, our bins, and vehicles all descended on the house at the same time. It had been thirty years since we had moved the last time and I was pleased at how well it went.

After the first week, the hospital suggested we take my father home on an outing so he could be away from the hospital for a day. The house was a mess at this point, boxes everywhere, and nothing organized, but I brought him to the home, so he could see the house and where it was.

He was exhausted by mid-afternoon and asked me to drive him back to the hospital and so I did. A week later the doctor called me to say they had released him just after we had left the hospital, so I turned around and picked him up. The staff told me he had made a miraculous recovery and that I was now his guardian and primary caregiver and so there I was with three people to look after full time.

It was easier with them living with us but we lost our privacy and my father was a bully all my life. He was always mean and it was hard for Hubbie to have him live with us, but at this point, we didn't have a choice. We never expected my father to move in with us because he was after all, going to be admitted to a nursing home.

My father fell down often in the house and in the yard and looking after him wasn't easy. He had a lot of doctor's appointments that year along with my husbands' appointments. I was beginning to lose my mind. I did not know if I was coming or going. I ended up buying a huge white board so I could keep track of all the appointments. I still rely on the board today it lets me keep things straight in my head on who needs to go where and when. We bought a baby monitor so we could hear when he woke up and could tend to his needs. He had a walker to help him get around the yard, but he hated using it. The bathroom in our bedroom has a shower, their bathroom had a bathtub, no shower. My father wasn't able to use the bathtub, getting in and out was impossible for him, so we let him use our shower. I ended up getting a bathtub handle and rigged a showerhead in their bathroom so my husband and I didn't have to share our bathroom with him. My mother was also using our shower and I did not understand why. She is healthy and capable of getting into a bathtub so we weren't sure why she wanted to use our shower, she hates showers.

There was a blizzard happening one day and my mother went to the fridge to get my father's insulin and looks at me and says he doesn't have any more insulin. I had to call the pharmacy and drive to town to get it. I wondered why she didn't tell me before-hand that he was running low on the insulin. It was one more thing I had to do, check on his pills and insulin and see when I should order them before he ran out. This happened twice before

I got a handle on it.

Emotions of the Year – Working Pages
That year my strongest emotions were: frazzled, losing my mind, pulling my hair out, short-tempered, and jealous.

Do you feel frazzled?
I was at my wits end. I had no time for me and it was all on me to do everything for my husband and my father. I actually needed the time to sit in a very hot bath just to relax.

I feel frazzled because:

_____

Do you feel like you're losing your mind?
I really did feel like I was losing my mind. Nothing made any sense to me and I felt so alone at this point. The only thing I had going for me was my strength to endure everything that was happening around me.

I feel like I'm losing my mind because:

_____

Do you feel like pulling your hair out?
There were days I just wanted to pull my hair out. People around me were being very stupid, saying things like I wasn't helping, or looking out for them, while all the time I was doing it for them. I wasn't sure what they wanted of me.

I feel like pulling my hair out because:

_____

Do you feel short-tempered?
Because of the things they were saying I snapped at people. I was cranky and felt bad because it wasn't their fault, so, I watched how I reacted to my husband, father, and mother.

I feel short-tempered because:

_____

Do you feel jealous?

Watching my husband and my father getting so much attention, I became jealous of them. I know it sounds stupid but I wanted to be looked after too. I got past it because I did not want to be sick but all the same it's what I felt at the time.

I feel jealous because:

_____

Tips from the Trenches

(TIP) Make the time for yourself. You will be of no use to your loved one if you don't do things you like to do.

(TIP) Get a white board to keep track of everything you do. It helps if your loved ones know what is happening. I listed doctor's appointments, when I ordered pills, and when I was picking them up.

(TIP) Get a baby monitor. I carried it with me at all times, that way I knew when my father woke up, so I could help him.

What I learned about myself…

I was and still am a very organized person, this I think, is my greatest asset. I accomplished so many things this year, I never thought I was capable of. Fear did not stop me from doing what I had to do to make my loved ones safe and well looked after. I was amazed at myself, how far I had come from the first days of being a caregiver to who I was now.

I was the primary caregiver and it seemed that I was enjoying it to the fullest even when some days were more difficult than others. I still went through the gamut of emotions but I was better at handling it now. I was stronger than I thought I was.

On the Lighter Side…

One day I was cleaning up around the property after a strong wind had knocked down branches and twigs the previous day. I was loading up the wheelbarrow and carried on. I went inside for a few minutes and when I came back out, I forgot all about the wheelbarrow.

At one point I asked my mother where my father was and she responded with, "I don't know."

I got concerned because now my dog was missing too. I called for her and she came running from the back of the property. There is a steep drop at the back and it is easy to fall down the slope if you're not careful.

I asked the dog what was wrong because she started barking at me and all I could think of was the line out of the show Lassie, "Lassie, what's wrong, is Timmy in the well?" I followed her and sure enough my father had taken the wheelbarrow to the back and slipped down the hill head first.

He was calling us but we couldn't hear him, he was too far away. After getting him out, we looked at him to make sure he was okay and saw he had ripped his shirt and pants, his hair was full of leaves and his knees were bleeding. Next thing I know my mother is getting mad at him for ruining his clothes and I was laughing because he really was a sight.

We helped him out and I told him never to do that again but it's pointless to tell him what he can or can't do. Needless to say, he was not allowed to help anymore but I thank our dog because she showed us where he was. My mother didn't see the humor in it but she wasn't about to watch what my father did or where he went.

"I was yelling for you", said my father. I explained that if you're two acres away nobody will hear you. He never understood that he was not allowed to go to the back of the property without proper supervision.

19 YEAR TWELVE – HOME ON THE RANGE

It was a relatively uneventful year regarding people being sick. I started to have some time for myself and it was great. I decided to take another University course.

We had settled into the new house and I began dealing with all the home issues, a new water system, new furnace, and a new roof. All that was required of me was to call someone and they would do the work, it was wonderful. I felt spoiled. It was such a nice feeling.

Mid-year my father needed a gall stone removed, so, I made sure he would get to the hospital for his appointment with his new doctor. This doctor should never have been allowed to be a doctor. His bedside manner was atrocious. He thought his time and his time alone was the only thing that mattered.

I took my course with me so that I could study while we waited. I could not believe the waiting time for this doctor to show up. On the first consultation, he made us wait for seven hours. My father hated waiting and I can't say I liked it much, but I stayed and the doctor finally showed up. I was truly annoyed with him. I even went so far as to tell him that my time was just as valuable as his. He did not care.

The surgery went well and they removed the gall stone without cutting into him and he was able to come home the same day.

I took my father in for the checkup after the procedure and once again I was furious with the doctor. I made the staff page him twice and told them I was leaving if he didn't show up in the next five minutes. The doctor did finally show up for the ten-minute checkup that turned out to be nothing, I left never to see that doctor again. I decided my fathers' family doctor could deal with anything else that was required because I refused to see such an arrogant doctor. I should have checked online to find out how that doctor rated with other people but I did not think of that at the time I talked to my father's doctor and explained the situation and said if he needs to see that type of doctor, he should give me a different one because I had better ways of wasting my time.

I enjoyed my summer that year, we had a lawn tractor and I mowed for hours. It was my safe place to go. I drove it around, mowing, and enjoying my alone time. I had time to think, my mind was at peace, and I was really calm. I looked forward to mowing twice a week. I had not met any of my neighbors at this point but as I was mowing one day, the guy next door got on his mower and met me at the fence and that was the first introduction.

Every time I got on the mower he would get on his and we would meet up and talk. I looked forward to mowing and one time I had shut the mower off and realized my neighbor was singing "Home on the range", while wearing his cowboy hat. He liked mowing just as much if not more than me. Mowing became better than having a bath or lighting candles. It was peaceful even over the hum of the engine and I looked forward to the next time I would be mowing. I was focused on the mowing, I thought of nothing else. I had no worries or thoughts of anyone else.

My neighbor asked my husband one time, "how much do you pay your wife to mow? Because she really looks like she's having fun." My husband's response was, "she won't let me use the tractor, she gets down right mad if I even suggest to mow".

My father was impressed I could run a lawn tractor. All my life he said women were useless and could never do a man's job. My mother always believed that but I never did.

I could do anything I set my mind to. Every time I mowed my father would come out and watch me mow.

Once when I was done mowing, he wanted to talk to me, I thought he needed something, but he just wanted to tell me that he was extremely proud of me for my accomplishments through the years. This was something I never thought I would hear. He couldn't imagine how I sold both properties and found a house we could all enjoy and be happy in together. I was speechless because he always put my mother and I down.

Again, after mowing, a few months later, he apologized for all the things he did to me my whole life. I didn't know what to make of that. We spent the afternoon talking and he looked remorseful for his behavior towards me while I was growing up. He never thought I could do all the things I was doing and had done throughout the years.

I never thought I would hear him say the things he said this year, never. It made me feel good and he continued to go outside every time I mowed to see me. I was now at peace with myself. I got my apology and praise, the thing I thought would never happen.

Being out in the country was everything I imagined and more. Life was looking up for me, it was fun. I learned to use a chainsaw and cut firewood for the fireplace. The property had a lot of fallen trees and I was able to clean up the dead wood and make the property what I wanted it to be like. I was busy and my mind got to recharge.

Emotions of the Year – Working Pages

That year the strongest emotions I had were: determined, surprised, enthusiastic, brave, and calm.

Do you feel determined?

I was on a mission to accomplish something that would make me feel good about myself again. Completing a university course would get me there and give me something to be proud of.

I feel determined because:

_____

Do you feel surprised?

I was startled at how well I was doing with my course and what I could do with my newly acquired hobbies.

I you feel surprised because:

_____

Do you feel enthusiastic?

I was on top of the world, I was able to look after everybody and still have time and energy to do what I wanted.

I feel enthusiastic because:

_____

Do you feel brave?

I now knew I could do anything that life threw at me. I could handle anything from this point on.

I feel brave because:

_____

Do you feel calm?

I was beginning to feel at peace with myself. I had a schedule and could look after everyone without feeling overwhelmed.

I feel calm because:

_____

Tips from the Trenches

(TIP) Find one thing you can focus in on that will require your full attention. It will help to think about something other than you already are going through.

(TIP) If you don't like the doctor you have, there is nothing stopping you from finding another one. Not every doctor is good or compatible with you. Only you know if the fit is right.

(TIP) Check out the comments section of the doctor you are about to see on the internet. This wasn't available when I was going through it.

What I learned about myself…

I would not tolerate fools. The doctor was arrogant and self-centered and I was not about to stand by and let him treat my father and me like that. My time was just as valuable as the doctor's and I told him so. I was now standing up for my rights and expressing my feelings when I was not treated properly. I never would have done that before but now it was a good feeling to have.

I was strong enough to confront the doctor and the hospital for their lack of common sense. No one should be treated badly no matter the situation. In the past I would never had said anything and now I was able to stand up for myself.

On the Lighter Side…

One day I was mowing when the tractor died. It yanked me out of quiet time. Of course, it died at the back of the property and not near the garage. I thought about what I should do. Should I try to push it up to the house? Or figure out why it died?

I wasn't going to be able to push it up the hill so I started hiking up to the garage. My husband showed me where he keeps the sprays, oil, and whatever else I might need in any situation. I remembered he told me he had a carburetor spray. Okay, I think to myself, it must be that afterall it would need a tune-up soon.

I got the spray and back to the tractor I went. I sprayed it and it tried to start but couldn't. I was getting upset because now I would have to wait for him to come home so he could help me. I hated asking for help.

When he came home, he went down to see what the problem was. He looked at me and said, "You're out of gas."

"DOH!!!" I felt so stupid at that moment, I forgot to fill up the tractor. All that fuss for nothing.

20 YEAR THIRTEEN – OH, LOOK, THE CANOLA IS BLOOMING, NOT!

2014 started out well but by spring everything became a nightmare once more. My father was once again feeling poorly and he was contemplating going to the hospital, but this time, he was afraid. I didn't understand because my father was never afraid to go before.

My father was very scared about having to go the hospital and this was out of character for him. In July he asked if I would take him and he had tears in his eyes. I became very frightened but I knew I he had to go to the hospital. He was admitted and I knew I would be taking my mother to visit him every day but that wasn't going to be a problem because she lived with us. No driving to pick her up.

We went to visit my father on a Saturday and he seemed to be doing well. My mother wanted to drive to the city to visit her friend after seeing my father and there was no need for her to be at home, so she went.

Friends were coming over that day and my daughter was with me because she too had gone to see her grandfather. The hospital called around noon and told me we needed to be there as soon as possible and I asked what had happened, the nurse told me she thought my father had passed away. I wasn't sure what that meant. Did he die or was he in his final stage of life? I was very confused. I tried to call my mother but I could not get a hold of her so I left a message. She finally called back and I explained to her that my father had passed away. My girlfriend would drive her to the hospital because my daughter and I left as soon as we got the call.

My mother could not handle dealing with the funeral arrangements, so again it fell to me. I took care of everything. That was the first time I ever arranged a funeral and I handled it magnificently. It all went well. The only problem with the funeral was my mother started screaming my father's name constantly. This coming from the person who didn't care about him and now she was showing some emotions. It was truly embarrassing.

My mother would not allow me to clean or mow or do anything, she wanted me to sit with her all the time. I asked my daughter to pick up my mother's friend and bring her out so I could do what I needed to do.

A few months had passed and now it was up to me to dispose of my father's belongings and I asked my mother if she was okay with it. We spent a week cleaning out his room and removing the furniture. It needed to be done at some point and I saw no reason to prolong it.

My husband suggested that I take the room and make it mine. I jumped at the chance. I never had a room that I could call my own and it was a great idea considering I had so many hobbies that were boxed all the time. It was a lot of fun unpacking and setting up all my hobbies. It was surprising to me that I had so many things I didn't have the chance to display before. Still today we go and look around the room and sit in it. It is such a happy room now and it has a great aura.

My daughter informed us that she was getting married in August and they wanted to get married on the acreage. Now the deck needed painting to look respectable and the yard pristine. After all, it was the first time she was getting married. There was a lot of work to do before the actual day. It was six weeks of hard work from the day my father passed away until the day she got married.

It took our minds off of losing my father with all the preparations required. I know I did more than I should have for the wedding but it was a distraction from mourning for my father. So, all in all, it was a rough year and again I came through it fairly well.

It was a busy eventful summer. Everyone complimented me on our property during the wedding, it was lovely to hear. The men barbecued and the women could sit around and chat. Near dusk, I started removing the steaks and burgers and someone commented that I was rude for taking the food into the house. My response was, look around, you will find there a many glowing eyes visible all around us in the bush. Coyotes smelled the food and I didn't think it would be good for people to get attacked. No one realized that there was wildlife all around us and before I knew it, everyone was going home, quickly, after my comment.

Emotions of the Year – Working Pages

That year the strongest emotions I had were: dread, disturbed, worried, uncertain, and alarmed.

Do you feel dread?

It became evident that my father would not be around much longer and I felt a cloud of dread hang over me. I did not know how to deal with it, so I tried to ignore the feeling. It didn't work, it was still there. I should have allowed myself to cry or talk to someone about what I was feeling but I did not.

I you feel dread because:

_____

Do you feel disturbed?

I had no idea what was about to happen or how I was going to handle it. I did not know how I would react if my father was gone. I was truly disturbed by my thoughts and I could not discuss it with anyone.

I feel disturbed because:

_____

Do you feel worried?

I became worried about my mother and how she was going to handle it if he passed away. They would have celebrated their 60th anniversary the following January.

I feel worried because:

_____

Do you feel uncertain?

It became a time of uncertainty for everyone. Nobody knew what was going to happen or when. I wasn't sure what to do or if there was anything I could do to help in this situation. It became a waiting game.

I feel uncertain because:

_____

Do you feel alarmed?

I was surprised at my mother because the way she was acting she couldn't care less if he lived or died. This, to me, was very alarming.

I feel alarmed because:

_____

Tips from the Trenches

(TIP) Do not bottle your emotions. It will only make you sick. Call someone, anyone.

(TIP) If you have a loved one in the hospital, call in advance to find out what things are acceptable to send in sympathy. Not all units accept flowers, for instance. The cardiac unit does not allow them. Only fruit baskets were allowed on the ward.

(TIP) If you are from out of town, the hospital will have a list of places to stay that are much cheaper than a hotel.

What I learned about myself…

No matter the situation, I could handle anything now. I had come a long way from who I was at the start of being a caregiver. I became assertive. I stood up to my mother for the first time and claimed my father's old bedroom even though she wanted it, she didn't need an extra bedroom, I did.

I could now be anything I wanted to be and I could conquer mountains if that was what I decided to do. I had transformed into someone I was proud of. It was a good feeling.

On the Lighter Side …

The farmers out here raise a lot of canola. It starts to bloom late July, early August. It's very pretty to see when you're driving. As far as you can see the farmland is covered in bright yellow.

In April of that year I took my father to the hospital because he wasn't feeling well. While I'm driving down the country roads my mother looks out the window at the side of the road and says, "Oh, look, the canola is blooming."

My father gets mad and says, "No, it isn't, that's a dandelion."

They got into an argument and I was going to be the judge. For the record neither of my parents listen to me or believe anything I say but I would have the deciding vote as to what was on the side of the road. I explained to my mother it couldn't have been canola because it was early April and the farmers hadn't begun to plant their fields yet. Now she was upset with me.

I couldn't stop laughing all the way into town. It really was a dandelion on the side of the road and I should have stopped so she could see what it was and she wouldn't be mad at my father or myself.

21 YEAR FOURTEEN – THE DAY I COULDN'T FIND MY PANTS

This year was the hardest year of all to cope with what was going to happen. It took everything I had in me to survive.

My husband had his yearly cardiologist appointment and were informed he developed A-Flutter. I had no clue what that was or what it meant. The doctor explained it and said my husband needed to be on blood thinners. The way his heart was working without blood thinners may cause him to have a stroke and also recommended he have a cardio-version done.

The doctor prescribed a new blood thinner that had just come on the market. We trusted him. The new blood thinner, unbeknown to us, had no counter agent.

When I was at home, I looked up information about A-Flutter and cardio-version. It wasn't very reassuring to me to find out what all that entailed. He was sick again.

The cardio-version was booked in for October of that year. It didn't seem so bad and he would go home the same day.

My husband developed an internal bleed that we were unaware of. He started getting dizzy and unstable. It became very scary, very quickly. Something was wrong. He was wobbling around, laying down most of the time, and developed nose bleeds during the night. I washed the sheets almost every day and tried to get out blood stains which are very difficult to remove.

In September I was keeping an eye on my husband because he wasn't doing so well. I was behind him when he almost went over the railing on the second floor. The steps leading up are divided with a landing half way up so the fall would have been half a staircase. I managed to grab him and pull him away. At this point, I told him to get dressed because he was going in to the hospital. Something was seriously wrong.

While we were at the hospital, I informed them that he was going to have a cardio-version at the end of October and could they not do it while he was there. Everyone agreed but when they checked him out, they said he was no longer in A-Flutter. Okay, that was good news.

His cardiologist worked out of the same hospital and I had called to tell him my husband had been admitted because of the bleed. He went to see my husband immediately.

The doctors told me he had lost six units of blood, more than half the blood in the human body. They gave me documents for the blood he received and said they didn't know if something would arise from all the blood they replaced, such as Hep C, or anything else. I was at a loss. This was very scary to me.

At the same time our septic tank fell apart and I took care of that on top of visiting him every day. I thought I was losing my mind at this point. How was I supposed to handle all of the crisis around me and still keep my sanity?

Our basement got flooded by the sump pump not working so I called insurance to see if they would cover the damage. They agreed to the cost so I had nothing to worry about.

I have a very nice gentleman that has handled our water system from the start and he informed me that I would have to remove the deck or they would not be able to fix it. Swell, remove the deck and visit my husband. My son-in-law, daughter, my girlfriend, and I, managed to take down the deck and I was ready for the septic tank repairs.

There I was, being my usual self and not thinking, just doing what was required. I, apparently, work well under pressure, and dealt with the home issues while still going to the city and seeing how Hubbie was doing.

The septic tank got was getting fixed but I asked my daughter if she could work from our house because my mother did not know what to do. There really wasn't much to do but wait for the job to be done and pay the workers. This wasn't hard but my mother couldn't even do that.

The insurance company packed up our basement and cut out all the damaged walls. It was a relief because I didn't have to do anything. I hated the basement from day one, so, this was my opportunity to find someone that would make the basement the way I wanted. We hired a contractor.

From September to the middle of November I had people in and out of the house doing everything. It was an inconvenience but it was all worth it. Our basement was transformed into the nicest room in the house and I was glad at how well and quickly it was done.

My husband remained in the hospital for three weeks and missed most of the activity coming from the house. It took the doctors all that time to figure out where the bleed was coming from and I was not about to take him home until he was once again okay.

I took him in for his cardio-version at the end of October and everything went well. My husband developed his A-Flutter again the following year but the doctor did not recommend the procedure again. We were told he would have to live with it for the rest of his life.

Emotions of the Year – Working Pages

That year the strongest emotions I had were: disillusioned, quitting, unfair, world to stop, unbelievable.

Do you feel disillusioned?

I was so disillusioned with the medical profession by this point. I did not trust them. I know why it's called practicing medicine, now. It was a guessing game for them.

I feel disillusioned because:

Do you feel like quitting?

This could not be happening to me. It was the worst year of all and I wanted no part of it.

I feel like I just want to quit because:

Do you feel life is unfair?

How could the medical profession fail us again? Why us? Will it never stop? It seemed like the world was being unfair to the both of us.

Do you feel you want the world to stop?

Whatever merry-go-round I was on, I wanted off. I did not want to go through this again. I wanted the world to stop but it wouldn't. Life goes on, as they say.

I feel like I just want the world to stop because:

Do you feel like this cannot be happening?

All I could think that year was, 'this can't be happening again'. How could this keep happening time and again? It needs to stop.

I feel like this cannot be happening to me because:

Tips from the Trenches

(TIP) Don't assume the doctors will give you the right medication. Find out more before just accepting it. I should have found out more about the blood thinner, but I didn't.

(TIP) Find a pharmacy you like. If they know you, they speed up the service. When my father was with me, the pharmacists would put together his medications immediately.

(TIP) Talk to your pharmacist about the medications you get, they will know about side effects or if there is a problem with it.

What I learned about myself…

I was no longer afraid of any problem that ensued in front of me. I just solved the situation and carried on with the next crisis. I let people help me. I no longer felt guilty if I wasn't the one fixing things. This was one of the hardest lessons I learned, before this I did it all myself rather than let people in to help. I always thought it would be a failing on my part if others were to help me.

On the Lighter Side…

One day when my daughter and I were going to visit her Dad in the hospital I couldn't find the pants I wanted to wear. I searched and I searched to no avail. I grabbed another pair and we were off.

While riding in the elevator with my daughter, another lady joined us. I looked at my daughter and told her I wasn't able to find my pants.

Now the lady in the elevator wasn't sure what to do after that comment. She looked uncomfortable after my statement. Yes, I was wearing pants but it wasn't the pair I wanted that day. What must have gone through this lady's mind and become tempted to look. Before we got to our floor the lady did look over and said to me, "You seem to have found them."

Yeah, still not the ones I wanted that day.

22 CONCLUSION

It has been a long and hard journey for me, but I made it. I am a completely different person now and it's been three years and everyone is doing great. I learned so much about myself through the years and what I'm capable of and I cannot see any barriers that could stop me from my future. I still remember everything I went through and how hard it was but I'm a better person for going through it.

In the near future I will be volunteering at a local hospital to help the elderly and possibly give workshops to the caregivers. I hope sharing my experiences as a caregiver will help others when they go through it also. No one talks about the caregiver and what they go through and I think it needs to be said. Today, with our parents living longer, there aren't enough nursing homes to accommodate everyone, so it's falling on the children's shoulders to care for their parents in their homes. We give up our careers, lives, and self-worth to do it. It needs to be talked about and be in the open so people are aware of it. Caregivers have feelings too. We need to talk about the problem's caregivers go through and what we can do to help other caregivers. It's important for caregivers to know there are people out there who can help.

A few years ago, Hubbie and I started walking slowly around our neighborhood and he no longer has A-Flutter and is doing exceptionally well. He is healthy and may be able to come off the blood thinners in the near future. My husband is a fighter and an inspiration to me every day. He never quits.

As for me, I spent fourteen years as a full-time caregiver for my family and I am still sane, not sure how, but I am. I look back at those years and can't imagine how I did it. I transformed into someone I thought I could never be. I look forward to a great and wonderful future. I realized that I too am a survivor.

Now the only person who needs my attention is my mother. She still leaves faucets running, pots boiling over, and fridge doors open. I find that this is not such a big deal because of what I did for so long and really, I just have to check around the house for anything she touches. She falls down quite often and because she lives with us, I need to get a caseworker to come in and assess the living arrangements and have it on file that she gets bruised when she falls. When my father was hospitalized the last time in his life, the hospital informed that it is better for me that he died in the hospital because if a death occurs in the house, I will be under investigation to find out if there was any elderly abuse happening. My mother is healthy and I assume that she will die in the house one day.

I am now a professional blogger and writer. I set up my website on my own and maintain it every day. I am extremely proud of myself. I have become a very confident and strong person. I can do anything I set my mind to. People enjoy reading about all the antics that happen in my life and I love writing about them. Never a day goes by when something unusual doesn't happen.

I have time to pursue all my old hobbies and found new ones I wanted to try. My life is now busy with fun activities. I learned to juggle in the past year, only to see if I could, before this, I couldn't even catch a ball and now I can catch three. I wanted to prove to myself I could learn a new concept and yes, I can. Now I'm in pursuit of new things to learn and do.

We also became grandparents and we are excited to spend as much time as we can with our little guy. We always wanted to have a grandchild and now we enjoy every moment with him. My grandson is the only one that will have a grandmother that can juggle because I don't think many people even considered it, why would they.

My life is very busy these days and I enjoy getting up every morning. I look forward to every sunrise and sunset but the stars at night are my biggest passion. My husband bought me a telescope but we haven't figured out how to use it, it doesn't come with instructions, and we can't find anything online that helps.

I've gone back to playing the piano, guitar, and flute. I relish my time playing music, once again. I didn't have the time during my caregiving days. I also returned to the treadmill and enjoy my one hour jog each day. When the weather gets better, I can jog around the neighborhood and I'm seriously considering entering running contests in the near future, to see if I can do it.

I discovered that I enjoy writing and I am now in the process of writing a science fiction trilogy for teens and I also enter writing contests.

Life is fun and I get to do what I want now and each day holds new opportunities for me and new discoveries about who I am.

23 WORKSHEETS

Do you feel angry?

_____

_____

_____

Do you feel scared?

_____

_____

_____

Do you feel frustrated?

_____

_____

_____

Do you feel like crying?

_____

_____

_____

Do you feel helpless?

_____

_____

_____

Do you feel hatred?

_____

_____

_____

Do you feel annoyed?

_____

_____

_____

Do you feel anxious?

_____

_____

_____

Do you feel sad?

_____

_____

_____

Do you feel hopeless?

_____

_____

_____

Do you feel grateful?

_____

_____

_____

Do you feel sorry?

_____

_____

_____

Do you feel elated?

_____

_____

_____

Do you feel good?

_____

_____

_____

Do you feel exhilarated?

_____
_____
_____

Do you feel unappreciated?

_____
_____
_____

Do you feel exhausted?

_____
_____
_____

Do you feel like withdrawing?

_____
_____
_____

Do you feel wiped?

_____
_____
_____

Do you feel you are being taken advantage of?

_____
_____
_____

Do you feel your life is a nightmare?

_____
_____
_____

Do you feel despair?

_____

_____
_____

Do you feel like you're living in hell?

_____
_____
_____

Do you want to scream?

_____
_____
_____

Do you want to hit something?

_____
_____
_____

Do you feel out of control?

_____
_____
_____

Do you feel depressed?

_____
_____
_____

Do you feel confused?

_____
_____
_____

Do you feel impatient?

_____
_____
_____

Do you feel overwhelmed?

_____

_____

_____

Do you feel relieved?

_____

_____

_____

Do you feel satisfaction?

_____

_____

_____

Do you feel proud?

_____

_____

_____

Do you feel impressed by what you did?

_____

_____

_____

Do you feel joy?

_____

_____

_____

Do you feel bad?

_____

_____

_____

Do you feel worthless?

_____

_____

_____

Do you feel sick?

_____

_____

_____

Do you feel tired?

_____

_____

_____

Do you feel fed up?

_____

_____

_____

Do you feel like running away?

_____

_____

_____

Do you feel like breaking something?

_____

_____

_____

Do you feel pity?

_____

_____

_____

Do you feel resentment?

_____
_____
_____

Do you feel detached?

_____
_____
_____

Do you feel stunned?

_____
_____

Do you feel inadequate?

_____
_____
_____

Do you feel unimportant?

_____
_____
_____

Do you feel distant?

_____
_____
_____

Do you feel anything?

_____
_____
_____

Do you feel frazzled?

_____
_____

Do you feel like you're losing your mind?

Do you feel like pulling your hair out?

Do you feel short-tempered?

Do you feel jealous?

Do you feel determined?

Do you feel surprised?

Do you feel enthusiastic?

Do you feel brave?

_____

_____

_____

Do you feel calm?

_____

_____

_____

Do you feel dread?

_____

_____

_____

Do you feel disturbed?

_____

_____

_____

Do you feel worried?

_____

_____

_____

Do you feel uncertain?

_____

_____

_____

Do you feel alarmed?

_____

_____

_____

Do you feel disillusioned?

_____

_____

_____

Do you feel like you just want to quit?

_____

_____

_____

Do you feel life has been unfair?

_____

_____

_____

Do you feel like you just want the world to stop?

_____

_____

_____

Do you feel like this cannot be happening?

_____

_____

_____

24 SELF CARE

I have included a few things to try. These may not be the things that will help you but it may trigger something inside you that you like doing. Everyone is different, try to make a list of some activities you enjoy and keep them close by to refer back to. I couldn't remember all of them at the time I was going through it but I did keep a list of a few of them with me at all times.

* Take a hot bath or shower
* Light some candles around the house
* Go for a walk, even if it's only for a few minutes
* Close your eyes and try to clear your mind
* Keep a diary
* Watch a show on TV that makes you forget about your life
* Meditate
* Take deep slow breaths
* Squeeze a stress ball
* Treat yourself to your favorite hot beverage
* Look outside and see the splendor
* Watch a bird or butterfly
* Stretch
* Do a crossword puzzle
* Aromatherapy
* Try to laugh about something
* Talk to a friend
* Cuddle with a pet
* Listen to your favorited music
* Get organized
* Do Yoga
* Clean a cupboard or closet
* Read a cartoon online
* Read a funny story online

Other ways to think about self-care are:

Using these 4 categories, think of something that makes you happy, makes you feel better, or gives you peace of mind:

Physical
* Things like going for a walk / run
* Doing Yoga
* Working out / going to the gym
* Dancing

Spiritual
* Prayer
* Meditation
* If you have a vocation or "calling", that activity

Emotional
* Having a good cry or laugh (maybe triggered by a sad / funny movie or story)
* Listening to music (though some might include that in spiritual instead / also)

Social
* Think of having coffee or a visit with your best friends
* Attend a support group
* Get involved in an online forum or chat group for caregiving

Another way to trigger ideas of self-care, still thinking of things that make you feel better:

What self-care things could you do if you had:
* 5 minutes
* 1 hour
* A whole day

Keep your list of self-care items somewhere you will see it daily, like on the fridge door. Whenever you are feeling low, and/or whenever you have a few minutes to yourself, visit your list and try to do at least one thing that will make you feel better.

Below is some space for you to write down your own self care items.

25 TIPS

(TIP) Anger produces energy. You can use that energy towards something constructive until it runs out.

(TIP) Try some deep-breathing exercises for a few minutes.

(TIP) Take a five-minute walk outside.

(TIP) Don't try to do everything yourself. Talk to someone. Check out what's available for you online. Cherish the good days, there will be a few in the beginning but as you go along there will be many more to come. Remember those days!

(TIP) Treat yourself to your favorite beverage or food. It will give you a short time-out.

(TIP) Phone or text a friend. They are always ready to listen and help and even if they don't, talking to someone that isn't going through what you are, helps.

(TIP) Taking a hot shower or bath will drain the tension out of your body and help you relax. If you like baths use Epsom salts or scented bubble bath.

(TIP) Enjoy a hobby if you have one. It doesn't matter how long you get to do it, but it does relax the mind doing something you like.

(TIP) When you're waiting at the pharmacy for medications, check out their pamphlets, there is a lot of information for caregivers.

(TIP) Strike up a conversation with a stranger and say a kind word to them you'll be amazed how much it will make you feel better.

(TIP) Look outside at the splendor in the world around you.

(TIP) Pat yourself on the back, you deserve it. No one else will but you can definitely feel good about yourself for being an amazing caregiver.

(TIP) Find a form of exercise, walking, jogging, or bicycling. It doesn't matter what it is but it will help your stress level go down.

(TIP) Listen to your favorite music or talk show.

(TIP) Read your favorite cartoon or comic strip, online.

(TIP) There will be situations that arise and sometimes you will need outside help. Don't be afraid to ask for it.

(TIP) Emergency responders know how to handle difficult situation better than you because you can't see it, you are the one going through it at the time.

(TIP) Use the hotlines in your area. You can find the number online. Where I live it's 811.

(TIP) Enjoy the down-time because you don't know how long it will last. Don't' waste a moment, embrace it. Do something that you enjoy whenever possible. You never know when the next crisis will occur.

(TIP) Squeeze a stress ball. You can find one anywhere, even the dollar store. I wore mine out.

(TIP) Petting an animal or playing with one lightens your mood.

(TIP) Don't forget to look after yourself. You're just as important as your loved one and you can't care for someone else if you get sick. Take care yourself, you'll be able to cope with the situation better.

(TIP) Get a Power of Attorney in place. The hospital may have some or else there are free ones online.

(TIP) Find out if you need a 'DO NOT RESUCITATE' (DNR), if that is what your loved one wants done.

(TIP) Find some humor in every situation you encounter. Laughter is still the best medicine.

(TIP) Make sure your loved one has a will or a living will in place.

(TIP) Check out monthly parking passes if it's going to be an extended time in the hospital. It's significantly cheaper
by the month.

(TIP) Don't go it alone. Use the resources available to

you.

(TIP) There are live chat lines online if you need to talk to someone anytime, day or night.

(TIP) Meditate if you can or do some yoga.

(TIP) Make the time for yourself. You will be of no use to your loved one if you don't do things you like to do.

(TIP) Get a white board to keep track of everything you do. It helps if your loved ones know what is happening. I listed doctor's appointments, when I ordered pills, and when I was picking them up.

(TIP) Get a baby monitor. I carried it with me at all times, that way I knew when my father woke up, so I could help him.

(TIP) Find one thing you can focus in on that will require your full attention. It will help you to think about something other than what you already are going through.

(TIP) If you don't like the doctor, there is nothing stopping you from finding another one. Not every doctor is good or compatible with you. Only you know if the fit is right.

(TIP) Check out the comments section of the doctor you are about to see, on the internet. This wasn't available when I was going through it.

(TIP) Do not bottle your emotions. It will only make you sick. Call someone, anyone.

(TIP) Find out if your loved one can receive flowers. The cardiac unit does not allow them. Only fruit baskets were allowed on the ward.

(TIP) If you are from out of town, the hospital will have a list of places to stay that are much cheaper than a hotel.

(TIP) Don't assume the doctors will give you the right medication. Find out more before just accepting it. I should have found out more about the blood thinner, but I didn't.

(TIP) Find a pharmacy you like. If they know you, they speed up the service. When my father was with me, the pharmacists would put together his medications immediately.

(TIP) Talk to your pharmacist about the medications you get, they will know about side effects or if there is a problem with it.

(TIP) Prioritize what is the most important thing to do for the day.

(TIP) Don't be afraid to ask for help.

(TIP) Keep a schedule.

(TIP) Plan ahead.

(TIP) Learn to say 'no'.

(TIP) Learn to do things more efficiently.

(TIP) Do not put off things you need to do.

26 ON THE LIGHTER SIDE: ENCORE

Wall Rash

My girlfriend was visiting one day and my husband was also at home and so was our daughter. I walked into the living room and promptly tripped, I still don't know what I tripped on to this day. My face hit the wall and wouldn't let go. I slid down the wall all the while trying to pry my face off to no avail. It felt like the wall had a suction cup in it and wouldn't release my face from it.

I didn't stop until I fell into the dog's food bowl, (I kept it in the living room because at the time my dog was blind and deaf), it was hard for her to get around. Now my face is covered in dog food and my dog was not amused, somehow, she knew I fell into her bowl. Trust me, I too was not amused.

At this point everyone was laughing their heads off, me, not so much. I was very embarrassed but I should be used it by now because I am the clumsiest person I know, but sadly I'm not. I fall down a lot, so much that I went to our family doctor and explained to her there is truly something wrong with me medically, there has to be a reason for this.

She made me go through many tests including bloodwork and told me I would get the results in a few weeks. I carried on as usual still falling down and hoping something would show up and explain why I'm so clumsy. I didn't want to be sick but at least I would have a reason for falling down.

The doctor called me into her office and promptly said, "there's nothing wrong with you, you appear to be just clumsy." Hmm, I think to myself, this is really bad, I have no excuse for my clumsiness now.

I left the office disappointed and starting walking home because the doctor's office was only a block away when I ran into a pole. I had a wall rash on the left side of my face and now I had a big lump in the middle of my forehead. That'll teach me. I guess the long and short of it is I lack concentration when I walk. By now you would think I knew how to walk but no I don't and over the years I still remain clumsy and continue falling down.

I do have days where I remain upright an entire day, but those are few and far between, and I wonder when strangers see me, they might think I am an abused wife but I'm not, my husband is a very kind and loving soul and not a mean bone in his body, but I still wonder if people think that.

Get Married to Each Other?

I cannot express the importance of getting out of the house. One time in our old neighborhood we decided to go to the corner pub. Everyone knows everyone. We lived in our house for over twenty years and a pub opened up. It was nice to have one because we could walk over and sit down with our neighbors and chat.

There was a lady that watched my husband and I sitting at our table and talking all the time. It was nice to be away from home and forget our troubles. We were unaware of her and she didn't come from our neighborhood but some of the neighbors knew her. She was reluctant to talk to us in case she disturbed us.

It didn't matter to us that it was a pub, if there was a restaurant in the area we would have gone there. We would have a pop or coffee and sit there for a few hours once or twice a week and enjoy the time we had away from home. We could relax and not think about work or bills.

One day someone asked me to come outside and show me their new vehicle. I gladly went and when I was done admiring the car when the lady that watched us came outside and began talking to me.

"I've been watching you two for some time and I have a recommendation for you." I could not imagine what she meant so I played along.

"What would that be?" I asked.

"You two should get divorced from your spouses and get married to each other", she says.

"What, no I don't think he'll marry me again?" I began to laugh and explained to her we are married but she wasn't getting it. "No, no, you should marry each other." No, no we are married to each other, really!

It took a while but she finally got it. She could not understand the fact that there were no other spouses involved. I told my husband and he found it funny because when we met each other decades ago we eloped in Las Vegas and nine years later we married again in a church. I wanted to be married in the eyes of God and he obliged. We never got a divorce but I did get married twice so it was humorous to us.

She had a hard time believing a couple could be married for that many years and still be in love as much as we were.

My husband still asks, "how many times do I have to marry you?" I would like to renew our vows on our fiftieth anniversary, so I guess the answer is three.

Dodging the Police

One day we decided to get on our motorcycles and cruise around town. My daughter was always thrilled to come along. When it came to being a passenger, she was amazing when riding on the back of her father's bike but at some point, she decided she preferred to ride with me. We didn't care which bike she was on and we loved having her with us.

With her Dad, she sat still and did exactly what she was told. On the back of my bike, that was a different kettle of fish. One time her running shoe melted on my exhaust pipe and she started moving around because her foot got a bit too warm and the bottom of her shoe had some bubble gum on it and was sticking. At the lights when we were stopped, I asked her what she was doing. Okay, no problem. I wasn't having any difficulty handling the bike.

We never discuss the route we'll take because my husband has no problems following me except once. I didn't realize the lights were going yellow, I did slow down and noticed a police car stopped at the lights across from us. I ran the yellow light and next thing I know the policeman puts on his lights and sirens.

I don't' know what went through my mind at the time but I started going down side streets in hopes of avoiding a ticket. Now my daughter is wondering what I'm doing and asks, "where are we going, do you know someone in this neighborhood?" she asks.

I stopped after I realized no one was following me. She indicates we've lost her Dad and he won't know where we are.

"First of all, your Dad knows where we live and can make his own way home and as for if we know someone around here, the answer is, no, I was dodging the cops."

My daughter began laughing and said, "Oh great, my Mom is teaching me how to get away from the police."

It might not be a lesson I wanted to teach her but what else could I have said. I didn't want a ticket for going through a yellow light. I do have a motorcycle license and am fully insured but I just didn't want a ticket.

My husband arrived at home before us and my daughter explained to him, Mom was dodging the cops.

What kind of an example I am to her?

Putting Together a Barbecue

I got tired of our old barbecue. One day I went out and got a new one. I thought I would help my husband out and put it together myself. What a big mistake, apparently, they're harder to assemble than I thought.

My daughter was visiting that day and she too wanted to put it together. We got out my tools and started the assembly. We were doing great until we got to the lid. It didn't fit. Hmm!!! For the life of us we couldn't figure it out. I was bound and determined to finish the job but there we were staring at a half-assembled barbecue.

We walked away from it and started to reread the instruction manual. It all seemed we did everything right but it didn't fit. At this point we both agreed that they gave us the wrong parts, what else could it have been? It never occurred to either of us that we may have done something wrong.

Again, we reread the instructions and decided we would start from scratch. Took it apart and put it back together. Nope, still didn't fit. Yup, must be something wrong with the parts, it couldn't be us, surely.

We struggled with it for hours and then my husband came home. He took a look at the barbecue and promptly told us to take it apart. My daughter and I looked at each other and told him, "they gave us the wrong pieces."

For the record, he was not impressed by us. He told us again to take it apart and then he says, "You put it together backwards."

Oh, is that the problem? No wonder we couldn't make it fit. Why would a company make parts that fit even if it isn't right?

So, there we were disassembling the barbecue and my husband told us to go away when we were done and let him put it together because obviously, we didn't know what we were doing.

We worked so hard that day to help him out so he wouldn't have to do it himself. Maybe it would have been better if we would have left it for him to do but we really did want to assemble a barbecue. Years later my daughter got a barbecue and managed to put it together by herself. Good girl!!! Way to go!!!

Me, I still don't' know how to put together a barbecue but in the near future, I will be replacing our old barbecue and maybe I will try again.

Buying a Juicer

My daughter's juicer died and she invited me to go with her. I was thrilled. We could spend a whole day shopping together. She juices fresh ginger for her migraines. She says it helps, but it became a problem when it stopped working.

We're out at a store and she begins her search. Not one of the juicers were the one she wanted. On to the next store we go. Someone working there asks if she could assist her and she asks for a brand of juicer and she says they don't carry that one.

Next store, again, no luck. At this point I'm starting to get annoyed. Does is really matter what kind it is? Apparently, yes it does. Off to the next store and the store person asks her if he could help. Again, that juicer is not available.

All of a sudden, she yells at me, "Come on, let's go, get into the car." We get into her car and she tells me that maybe she shouldn't have yelled at me in the store. I thought nothing of it at the time because I knew she was getting annoyed at not finding the juicer she wanted.

So, I asked her why she shouldn't have yelled at me and she says the store could call social services on her and accuse her of elderly abuse. I started laughing. I don't think I would classify that as elder abuse, really. We all get annoyed sometime and it was frustrating for her but it would have been hilarious if social services arrived while we were shopping.

I get into the car before her and when she gets in, she asks me why I was helloing her. Uh, what? I wasn't saying hello at all I was just sitting in her car waiting for her to drive to the next store.

Ok, now I think I should be worried. My daughter is hearing voices and it wasn't me. I was being as quiet as a mouse. I sure hope she doesn't get dementia before me because that might be an issue down the road.

Camping

We were camping at a national park after my husband's first heart attack. We took our motorcycles and this was the longest ride I was ever on. I was exhausted but pleased with myself for getting there.

The next day we wanted to explore and see the sights but I did not want to drive in the town. I'm good for highway riding but cities are another thing. We discussed it and both of us agreed I would ride on the back of his bike.

It was a long time since I was a passenger so we took it easy. We rode up a mountain and I was enjoying the scenery when I saw a sign on the side of the road. "Please keep your arms and legs inside the vehicle." Ok, here's the problem, where am I supposed to put my hands? I was holding onto my husband and there is no 'inside' on a motorcycle. Now I'm getting worried. What if a bear did decide I would be his lunch? It wouldn't be difficult for a bear to grab me and take me away.

We reached our destination and ate our lunch at the hotel on the top of the mountain. I asked my husband if he saw the sign about keeping your limbs inside the vehicle and he promptly started laughing. I did not see the humor in it but then he says it's the old saying, 'I don't have to outrun the bear, I just have to be faster than you.

Oh great, so many comedians out of work and I am married to one! I don't think he realizes it but I can run faster than him now. Wouldn't he be surprised?

Easter Eggs

Ever since my daughter was in elementary school one of her teachers got them to color Ukrainian Easter eggs. When she got home, she told me all about it. I was helping out at school every day so I went to her teacher and asked what I needed for coloring these eggs.

I drove downtown and purchased everything required from a Ukrainian Store. Since that first year we make Easter eggs on Good Friday.

First off, I need to tell you my countertops are made of granite in this house. The second year of living here we were coloring eggs and my daughter was doing an amazing job. It was the best egg ever, it was beautiful.

I was at the sink looking out the window and my daughter tells me to look at her egg. Before I could turn around, I heard a crack. Oh dear, that didn't sound good. What happened?

My daughter says, "I think I broke it." I look at her and the egg and felt bad for her. it did break on the counter but then she decides to poke it to see if it really was broken and she tells me, "yup, now it truly is broken."

Why on earth did she poke it? It may have been salvageable before that. I could have sprayed it with a varnish and all would be well, but no, she just had to poke it and make it worse. After the initial shock she started again but this time it wasn't as nice as the first egg. Too bad!

Every year since then, I cover the island with thick heavy towels to ensure it will never happen again and it hasn't. if only I knew back then, because it was such a professional looking Easter egg and she has never done such a lovely job on any other egg.

Moose in the Yard

Our first year living in the country was an eye-opener. Our dog was definitely a city dog. She was not accustomed to wildlife in our yard.

One morning I let her out in the yard to do her business when she high-tailed to the back part of the yard. I knew she went to chase whatever was there so I ran to stop her. Do not mess with the wildlife!

I caught up to her and almost ran into a family of moose. Just for the record, when you see the antlers up close you really don't want to be there. So, there I am, staring at the family of moose and I notice my dog racing to the back door and leaving me to deal with the situation.

I remembered what the park rangers told me if I came across a bear and I thought I would try it. I didn't look at the moose in the eye but I looked down and began saying, "please don't hurt me Mr. Moose, I'll just walk away." All the time talking to him I started walking backwards towards the house. Never turn your back on wildlife under any circumstance.

This was our first year in the house and there are a lot of trees everywhere. I didn't know my way around yet. So, there I am trying not to back into a tree or trip on a stump and talking to the moose. Luckily, I managed to get back to the deck without getting skewered. Yay me!!!

The moose are quite tame out here and are used to humans being around but at the time I didn't know that. Later I started thinking about what my dog did. Aren't dogs supposed to protect their humans? Mine apparently, thought about saving herself then and ran back to the house leaving me to fend for myself. Man's best friend, I think not!

148

Power Outage

When we moved out here, we needed internet, afterall we have a computer business and need access to it at all times. I got a local internet provider and all was well for some time. They put an antenna on our roof, which was rather tall, five feet high. It needed to be taller than the trees but it wasn't. The antenna worked on radio waves and every time it was windy it wouldn't work.

I called them every time and they would come out and look at it and try to make it work. one day when it was windy, I heard a big bang and investigated what the noise was. Nothing in the house was askew so I went outside thinking maybe a tree fell down. No trees were down and then I look at the roof and sure enough I noticed the antenna fell off. Back on the phone I go. They come out and this time secured it better than the first time.

For every phone call I made to them, they would try to remedy the situation. They never tired of my calls but we were frustrated not having internet. One time they came out and told me we had to cut down some of the trees. I would gladly oblige if it would fix the problem. I explained I would cut them down immediately when one of the guys said he would cut them down if I had a chainsaw. I just happened to have one and I notice he's having way too much fun and I wasn't. I like using the chainsaw but I didn't get the chance that day, too bad. He had a great time doing it and thanked me before leaving.

Next time I called, I told them we were having problems again all weekend. I explain the problem and while talking to him the power goes out and the phone goes dead. I grab the phone that works even in a power outage and call him back. I apologized for my rudeness because my phone went dead.

He tells me to check the speed I'm getting on the internet and realizes what he said, "call me back when the power comes back on." I don't need to wait because my computer is on and still running.

"I'm sorry ma'am, if the power is out you cannot access the internet."

"Yes, I can."

"No ma'am, your computer cannot work without power."

At this point, he doesn't believe me and thinks he's talking to one stupid woman. I get it, it does sound stupid but then I explain, "we have a UPS (uninterruptable power supply) on each of our computers" for just such an event. They will work for about an hour before the battery runs low, just enough time to finish what we're doing before turning them off.

Here this guy thought he was talking to a dummy but I am smarter than the average bear!!! So there!!!

Car Wash

We've all been to the automatic car washes at one time or another. My mother refuses to drive my vehicle if it's dirty so I make a point of washing it all the time.

I go to one car wash in particular because it does a really good job. The car wash has a bar indicating the maximum height, this way you know if your vehicle is too tall and one just at the entrance of the wash. If your vehicle touches the bar one should turn around and not proceed forward.

I'm at the car wash and there's a long lineup, five cars ahead of me. The vehicle just in front of me went past the first bar and I think nothing of it. We get to the front of the line and he proceeds into the wash. I'm sitting there watching when his vehicle starts going inside and he hits the bar. He has a Thule on top of his vehicle and next thing I know the bar is squashing his Thule. I have never seen anything like this before.

He keeps on going in and I get it, it's too late for

him to backup but he had to have hit the first bar. Why did he not stop then? He pushes through but the car wash does not engage and he gets to the end and now his Thule is crumpled in pieces, parts were just dangling and waving in the air. Now, where the dryer is his Thule begins to demolish the dryer vents. He destroyed the dryers and I have no hope in drying my vehicle when I get there.

He finally gets out and there is a breeze and his Thule is broken and the dryers are mangled. I managed to get my car washed that day but it was a sight to see.

The next time I go to the wash a sign is up, 'car wash down for repairs. No kidding!!!! What a moron.

Now when I pass the car wash, I always say, "Please don't break my car wash." I don't know how much these Thule's cost but I imagine they're not cheap. Whatever possessed this guy to carry on after the first bar? Moron!!!

Replacing Brakes

A few years after my husband's bypass, he figures his head is back and he can replace my brakes. I'm pleased to know I won't have to pay out too much money for a brake job. He used to do minor repairs on the vehicles before his first heart attack.

My girlfriend asks if her husband can park his motorcycle in our barn because they're having repairs done on their house and they need room in their garage. No problem, we have lots of room because we have a barn at the back of our property. We keep our bikes in the barn and we have bicycle stand (used for tuning up our bikes in the spring), tools, our bicycles, and our motorcycles.

My husband drives my van to the barn and decides to make more room, so he moves our friend's bike from the center and drives our bikes to the driveway in front. All is safe. He's gone most of the day and I start to worry. It never took that long before and I think maybe something has gone wrong. I went and checked on him and he starts telling me about everything that happened.

"I forgot when you replace brakes you must pump the brake a couple of times before doing anything."

I have no idea what that meant but I listen to his story.

"I turned on the van and stepped on the gas and I had no brakes. I finally figured it out but I managed to run into my bike stand before I stopped."

Luckily, he moved the bikes before because if our friend's bike was parked where it was originally, we would have to do repairs on it. He tells me he's going to glue his bike stand and all will be well. Yeah, no!!! All the glue in the world could not fix it. it was bent and out of shape and broken.

Well, on the upside, I have three brakes replaced because he couldn't get the fourth brake off. Now when I stop at lights that brake squeaks very loudly all the time. My husband still hasn't got the courage to try again.

I was lucky that day that he didn't go through the back of the barn. Can you imagine what it would have cost? A new barn, a new bike for our friend, and a bike stand. In the end my husband finally broke down and bought a new bike stand, he gave up with the glue, eventually.

Stupid Slippers

I took my mother up to get her eyes checked and in the same strip mall is a store that carries unique items. When I'm there I always check it out.

We're in the store and I spot the cutest slippers so I buy two because they're cheap and I like them.

I bring them home and put on a pair. It's Friday and date night in the basement. I'm wearing my new slippers and I head for the basement, as I'm going down the stairs I slip and fall. I don't think anything of it because I am clumsy. Okay, so it's pill time and I go upstairs to get my husband's pills and treats for the animals. I start going up and trip again. Now this is starting to annoy me, I hurt my arm and shoulder the first time and now my shins are hurt.

The evening is over and we head to bed, as I start climbing the stairs to our bedroom, what should happen? I trip before the landing and my head hits the wall. Ow, I look and now I have managed to put a dent there and my head hurts.

Next morning, I look at the wall and discover it's not too bad. I get a plaque and cover it up until I can repair it. No big deal and never mind I have a lump in the middle of my forehead.

I realized I hurt all over and figure out it's all because of my new slippers that I kept on falling. I get the slippers and promptly throw them in the garbage. What a waste, they were just so cute but I was a menace wearing them.

Now, every time I go upstairs, I'm reminded of that day because I can see part of the dent, the plaque does not cover the entire damage, apparently my head is bigger than I thought it was.

So, needless to say, I'm back to wearing my old slippers.

Baby Gates are Hazardous to your Health

When we move into our house our basement was awful and one day, I would remodel it. The people that owned the house before us let their dog use it for a toilet. I steam cleaned it when we moved in but the odor was still there.

Our dog would go downstairs at night if she had to go to the bathroom and I became annoyed at that point so I bought a baby gate and put it up every night. At that time our office was in the basement and I don't want the smell of urine all day. I managed to get it clean after several cleanings and the smell was gone.

One night, after date night, my husband tries to put up the baby gate and cannot manage it. I figure I can do it, so I push him out of the way. He gets annoyed with me and tells me fine you do it if you're so smart.

I know I can, I've done it before. Never, ever, think you can do it better than anyone else and here's what happened. I struggle with the gate and before I know it, I'm sliding downstairs on top of the gate. I ended up stopping on the landing and ramming my head into the wall.

I stay like that for a few minutes and then my husband says, "that's going to hurt." No kidding!!!

The next morning, I look at the wall, no damage, yay but my head hurts and a lump has appeared, really no big deal, I'm used to it. My gate is now in pieces and I figure I can fix it. I got plastic ties and glue and it looks like it will stay together and so it does. I have yet to replace it and it has been several years, so that's good.

I don't know what possessed me that evening to take over and do it myself. Now I wish I had a normal flight of stairs without a landing because generally there is no wall at the bottom that close to the stairs but sadly, both my staircases have landings and I will continue to run into them at one time or another.

Lesson learned, do not try to show off to your husband that you can do it better than him. Nothing good will come of it. On the upside, I now know what it's like to slide down the stairs. Whoopee!!!

Choking on Coffee

I swear I'm going to buy myself a sippy cup. Somehow or another I choke on the coffee while drinking it. By now you would think I knew how to drink liquids.

I was in the office and took a sip of my coffee

when it goes down the wrong hole. I'm sure it's happened to everyone once, to me it happens all the time. I started choking and ran to the bathroom sink. I cannot for the life of me catch my breath, only short little ones and now I'm wheezing and coughing. This goes on for at least a half hour.

My mother is heading downstairs and pays no attention and my husband is in his bathroom staying away. No one comes to help or see if I'm okay. Everyone has vanished, no one to pat me on my back or anything. I stay in the bathroom hacking by myself.

After I get over this episode I go downstairs and my mother says, "what happened to you?" Really, that's what you say? You could have tried to help, but no, why would you? I hate to tell her if something happens to me, I don't think my husband will let her live with him without me there, so there.

Now my husband comes out of his bathroom and looks at me and says, "sounded like someone was hoarking up a lung." Yes, that was me.

I recovered from that and finally ask why he didn't come help if he could hear there was a problem and he always came up with the same answer, "I know you, you always have it covered."

Seriously, you're not a big help in a crisis!!! I must keep telling myself, do not rely on anyone for any help ever. Sheesh!!!

A few months later I find out my girlfriend has never choked on anything. Hmmm, maybe it's just me? Oh dear!!! A sippy cup it is!!!

Getting Clocked
When we moved in here the fireplace is huge and a nail sits in the middle of the stones. Wonderful, I can put a clock there. There's only one problem, I'm short and I need a ladder to get it up there.

155

One day I notice my clock has stopped. No problem, I'll just replace the batteries and all is right again, problem. I couldn't reach it and I didn't get out the ladder. I couldn't reach out but I figure I'll get the tongs from the kitchen and get the clock down.

It wasn't working very well the tongs weren't strong enough but I was bound and determined to accomplish this feat. I struggled and struggled. The tongs finally caught and the clock was coming down. I realized the clock was falling down so I tried to grab it with my other hand. It hit my head and bent my glasses. I wear progressives and if they are out of alignment the world just doesn't look right and I get dizzy looking through them.

Now, I figure I need to go to my optometrist to get them straightened. I sat down to wait and when the lady comes out and takes one look at me and tells me to give her my glasses. Wow, she figured out my problem without me telling her.

She brings them back and asks what happened because they were really out of whack and it must be hard to see anything. I agreed and told her my story.

"Well, you see, I was trying to get the clock off of the fireplace, it slipped, I got my head to stop it, and knocked my glasses out of alignment. Essentially, I got clocked in the head with a clock."

Now everyone in the office starts laughing at my expense and I decide to laugh with them. Why not? It was funny.

I go back every year and each time I go in they start laughing, too bad they still remember me and my story. I've been told I'm a very memorable person. Yeah, right, I wish people would remember me when I do something normal but I guess that's not my lot in life.

Bookcases

I am an avid reader and amasses a lot of books.

When we moved in here my husband decided he would build me a bookcase in the basement. First off, my husband is not very good at carpentry but I wasn't about to stop him. He put up a bookcase and now I could have all my books available whenever I wanted.

Our office was in the basement too. I had my desk and computer right beside the bookcase and thought nothing of it.

A few months later I heard a creak and didn't pay any attention to the sound. It kept getting worse and I should have been alarmed but I wasn't. We were both at our desks working away and suddenly the bookcase fell apart.

There I was with piles of books all around me, on me, and on my desk. My husband does not respond to it, he just sits there. After a few minutes it occurs to him what happened. The books hit my head, which really, by now, I'm used to my head getting in the way.

He gets up and looks at the situation and it finally occurs to him maybe he should try to clear off some of the books. I just sit there, stunned, books are heavy when they fall on you and I look and start clearing away the books. We placed them in piles on the floor and my husband informs that maybe he should have built the bookcase better. Ya think???

After that he decided to make a better bookcase, one made out of wood, and no brackets with weak metal.

It never ends for me but why does it always happen on my head? My head isn't that big!!!

Dog Fight

Our dog went through an operation and she was overweight. We started taking her for walks again. She was doing great but needed to lose some of the weight she gained before her operation.

We were walking down the road and I saw

another dog in the middle of the road. I stopped and told my husband the dog was going to attack you could just see it. He doesn't believe me but I turned around with our dog and next thing I know the strange dog is attacking and at this point I'm trying to get the dogs apart. Meanwhile, my husband is walking slowly, very slowly, back towards us. No big help I must say.

I grabbed the stray dog and pulled but I fell down and found it difficult to pry them apart.

My leg really hurt the next morning and I assumed it happened when I hit the pavement. Nope, when I looked at it, it was a dog bite. I did not feel it because of the adrenalin rush you get while defending your own, at the time. Now I don't know if it was my dog or the other one that bit me during the altercation. All I know is that I came out of the dog fight the worst for wear. That was a first for me, being in a dog fight and also getting bit. Now, I think to myself, 'you should see the other guy', yeah, no, I was the other guy. Dogs are fine, me, not so much.

Now my dog refuses to go with us, not happening. You can just see it in her face, as if to say, 'are you nuts, it's dangerous out there'. She stays inside and waits for us to come home, and is quite content, all warm and happy.

Getting Skunked

Friday nights are always date night in the basement. We play pool, listen to music, and talk. One night were downstairs and I get a whiff of something. I tell Hubbie that it smells like a skunk and I start to worry. Did a skunk get in the house? Next thing I know my mother is yelling from the living room.

I went upstairs to check on her and the stench was incredible. It definitely smelled like skunk. My mother says she saw a dog at the window and next thing that happened was the smell.

She tells me to look outside. I think not!!! You go look if you're that curious, I am not. If there is a skunk under the window and I open the door I'm pretty sure I'm going to get sprayed and I don't have enough tomato juice in the house to wash myself with, at least that's what I heard gets rid of skunk odor from the skin. I'm smart enough to know when to go and look and when not to but if she wanted to find out if there was a skunk outside, she could look. Chances are if she did, I wouldn't let her back inside.

I felt sorry for the dog at that moment but I really felt sorry for us. How do we get the smell out of the house? Do I need to wash the entire house, walls and all, with tomato juice?

There was no hope! It's not like I could go outside and breathe fresh air or open the windows and doors. The skunk was right outside the front door and I figured if I opened the front door the skunk would get startled and that would make it even worse. Did not want the skunk to spray anymore, once was enough.

And so, there we were on Friday night with the odor of skunk all around us and us trying to have a good evening. Not!!! Have you ever tried playing pool when your eyes are watering so bad you can't see, well, that was us, what a sight! Okay, not a sight, because we couldn't see anything.

After a few hours it started to dissipate and we could start to breathe and see again. Yay us! I'm thinking we should get oxygen masks for just such an occasion. Hope they have ones for cats and dogs because the odor gets into your throat and you can taste it for a long time.

We can still get a whiff of it every now and again, inside and out, but it's getting better. How long does this smell linger, I'm wondering? So, on Friday night, all I can say is, "WE GOT SKUNKED".

Cold Medicine

Last year I caught a bad cold and thought I would get a hot lemon drink for my cold, (generic). Did not read the package. I drank my hot lemon drink and felt way better! About an hour later I wanted another, drank it and was now feeling on top of the world. What a bad mistake!!! I wanted another but I stopped myself. My daughter came by for a visit and I told her all about feeling great and she says to me, "I think you might want to consider joining a support group. You sound like you're hooked on it. You might need some help", she says.

But why, it helped me feel much better. Yup, and that was the problem, I wanted more. She says to me, "Hi my name is Alexa, and I'm an addict, its been (insert length of time here), since the last time I had my lemon drink.

You get the picture. I thought it was really funny at the time.

So, now I could picture myself standing up and saying, "Hi, my name is Alexa and its been three months, six days and fourteen hours since my last lovely hot lemon drink."

Now, I caught another cold and I keep looking at the box containing my cure for the common cold in the pantry and have to stop myself from taking one. Who knew it was addictive? It's only a lemon drink for heaven's sake! Yesterday my daughter and her family come over because my son-in-law has to winterize their camper and she starts to remind me of what happened last year with my cold. "Don't do it", she says. Ahh, come on, it made me feel way better last year.

I'm not finding it very funny today because I still have some and think to myself, should I, or shouldn't I have some. I am so tempted but alas, I will not.

What do they put in it? I wonder? I start to read the package and it says if you are diabetic, do not drink it. Oops, at the time I was diabetic, I'm not anymore but at the time last year, I was. One should always read the label before consumption. Silly me!!!

So, for now, "Hi my name is Alexa, and it's been twelve months, two weeks, and twelve hours since my last episode of a hot lemon drink."

This Is My Gene Pool???

There are some people who won't even try to do things for themselves. My mother is one of those people. This week I had to do a lot of things for her. She doesn't even try.

On Saturday evening Hubbie and I were relaxing and enjoying our time together when all of a sudden, my mother starts telling me I have to fix her clock.

All it needed was a new battery. How hard is that to replace a battery, apparently harder than one would think. Open flap, take out old battery, put in new one, and voila, clock works.

She tells me she's so impressed I can fix things. That's not fixing it in my opinion.

A few days later she yells at me to come downstairs, and so I do. I honestly thought it was an emergency. She says to me, "Is this a left—handed can opener?" Say what? There is no left-handed can opener available, as far as I know. I am a left-handed person living in a right-handed world and I don't know if I could use a left-handed can opener. That would be just weird.

She put the can opener on top of the can sideways and said it didn't work. No, duh!!!

I show my mother how to do it, put the opener on the side of the can and turn the knob. Now she is truly amazed. I think she does it on purpose just to make me do everything for her.

"Come to the bathroom" she says, "there's no hot water". I look at the problem, "next time maybe you should turn on the hot water tap?" I said.

When is the long weekend, what's on my wrestling channel, how do I turn on the microwave, how do I turn on the washer? These are the things I get asked all the time. It doesn't matter what I am doing at the time but I must fix the problem every time.

This week she decides that she was going to wash her floor and not ask me. Yay! I leave her to the task at hand. I was walking past and realized she was using my Vileda backwards. She is spraying herself and pushing the Vileda really hard.

This is my gene pool??? I explain to her that she is using it backwards and I actually had to show her how to use it. I would have thought that if my pants were getting wet that I was doing something wrong, wouldn't you?

Oh, yes, and yesterday she asked me how to use her heating pad. One must plug it in first and then set the temperature. "It only has one temperature", she says. No, I'm pretty sure it has – low, medium, and high. I showed her that you push the button up or down and see more temps.

"Which side of the pad do I use?" Yikes!!! "Why don't you put your hand on it and see?" I was pretty sure both sides get warm and they do.

It's a good thing my mother doesn't know how to use a computer because I don't think she would be impressed with me writing about her, but it's all true.

If I get that stupid when I'm her age, I've already told my daughter to put me in a home. What's the point?

This truly is my gene pool! I'm sticking with, 'I'm adopted'.

Soliloquy

We were sitting at the bar table in the basement one night, talking. My husband decides he's going to ramble on and I sit there listening. At some point I don't remember what happened but when I came to, I found myself lying on the floor.

While I was on the floor, I asked my husband what happened and he explained to me that I fainted. I crumpled up and fell off the bar stool. These bar stools are four feet off the ground, taller than most bar stools. I got up and realized everything on the table came with me. Now the carpet is stained and I run upstairs to get my cleaning products and start scrubbing the carpet. Stupid!!! It could have waited until morning but I'm just a stickler when it comes to stains and dirt. I must do it immediately.

This was the first time something like this happened. I've never fainted before and don't want to ever again. The next day my husband wants to know what happened. I have no idea! How would I know because it's never happened before? I don't know why either.

A week goes by and my husband finally says to me, "I'm not happy that you fainted during my soliloquy but now I can't remember what I was talking about." Oh, good because I don't want a repeat performance, really!!!

Did he really think I did it on purpose? Maybe that will teach him, do not keep going on and on because obviously I got so bored, I fainted. Now the jokes on him and he's worried about me for a change. Still to this day his side of the conversation is much shorter and I get a chance to talk too. I have no idea what he was talking about that night and it doesn't matter, does it?

I went to my doctor to find out why this happened and now I am going to go through a battery of tests over the next while but I realized I lost 'my big girl status', because my husband is now going in to the doctor's office with me. I am not allowed to go by myself anymore, he wants to make sure I tell the whole truth. Oh great!!!

Pool Balls Explode???

We were playing pool the other day and well, my husband always wins the majority of the games. All of a sudden, he exclaims, "Did you see that?"

"See what?"

"The ball moved."

"No, duh! You took a shot", I say. If one hits the white ball the balls move. It's not that hard a concept. I had no idea what he was trying to say to me.

"No, it moved before I took my shot", says my husband. "I swear, it really did move."

Seriously? I'm not sure what to make of this. Is the pool table now suddenly possessed? Or maybe, the balls? I, think not! I never saw the ball move until after he took his shot, but I believe every word he says, so, who knows, maybe it did.

Or, maybe, we have ghosts in the basement, or maybe there was a gust of wind? I can never distinguish if my husband is being serious or he's just pulling my leg. No, he was being serious. Huh!!! Well, it's better than the days in the 1800's. Pool balls used to explode.

Back in 1869 pool balls were made out of celluloid, an unpredictable plastic. As one took a shot and the balls hit each other small explosions would occur. Who thought that was a good idea? What fun that would be watching the ball explode!

I read an article that mentioned back then that when a ball would explode it wasn't out of the norm for the men to pull out their guns because it sounded like a gun shot. I'm not sure I would have liked to play pool back then.

I'd be putting my hands up in the air and surrendering too often. My arms would get tired, no?

And back in that day they also made lady's combs, buttons, collars, and dentures. Whoa!!! Can you imagine having dentures that were highly flammable and may cause a mild explosion in your mouth?

I would worry about having dentures like that. I fall down a lot so, when I fall my teeth smack together and boom, I would have exploded. Okay, my mouth would have lit up. Ouch!!!

Oh, look, my mouth is on fire! Oh, no, wait my button exploded. My wife's hair is on fire! What does one do in that situation, exactly? It must have been a very dangerous life to lead. You would not know when you might catch fire.I don't think I would have ever opted for false teeth, would you?

These are all actual events that happened to me or around me. Never a week goes by that nothing happens. I still fall down, choke, or hurt myself. I don't think I will ever lead a normal life. I've learned to laugh at myself all the time. Life is fun if you choose to look at it that way, life is too short to be serious all the time. When I was young, I was a very serious child and I never laughed. Today, I laugh all time even through a crisis because if you don't you will go crazy. There is never a dull moment in my life and it will probably continue to be that way.

There are a lot of good days, fun days while being a caregiver, all you have to do is look. I still remember them and laugh. It wasn't all bad. Life has a way of going on even if you don't want it to, so make the best of it, always. Take one day at a time and don't sweat the small stuff. Focus on today and not tomorrow.

27 RESOURCES

This website will give you all the information needed to find a support group nearest you or you can talk to them online if you live in the **United States.**

https://www.caregiver.org/support-groups

This is the **Canadian** website which will direct you to all the information you will need including support groups in your area.

https://www.comfortlife.ca/retirement-communities/caregiver-resources

For each city there is a different hotline you can call if you want to speak to someone in person. There are too many for me to list here but check online for the number in your area.

Check out doctor's offices, optometrists, and pharmacies for pamphlets. I was truly astounded to find so much information on caregiving.

Look online, there are chat lines on the internet if you want someone to talk to at any time for caregivers.

Your friends and family may have suggestions also or maybe able to help.

Caregivers burnout –

https://www.caregiver.org/depression-and-caregiving

https://www.caregiver.org/depression-and-caregiving

https://www.caregiver.org/caregiver-depression-silent-health-crisis

https://www.caregiver.org/caregiving-spouse-–-social-emotional-and-physical-issues

https://www.aarp.org/caregiving/life-balance/info-2017/spouses-marriage-stress-bjj.html

https://www.mayoclinic.org/healthy-lifestyle/caregivers/in-depth/caregiving-and-marital-strain/art-20114470

Other places to visit for a daughter/son looking after his/her parent/parents:

https://www.whereyoulivematters.org/role-reversal-like-become-parents-caregiver/

https://caringpeopleinc.com/blog/caregiving-parent-roles-reversed/

https://www.crosswalk.com/family/parenting/coping-with-role-reversal-more-adults-caring-for-aging-parents-11538630.html

There are so many articles out there that talk about what we go through as a caregiver but they all say the same thing. Look after yourself. No matter what the situation is, it is about giving yourself some time to recharge and carry on.

Role-reversal happens over time even when you didn't expect it and there is nothing you can do about it in some cases but to learn to live with it.

Documents you will need for the hospital.
Canada:

http://www.truehelpinternetwork.com/freelegalforms

United States:

https://formswift.com/

Enduring Power of Attorney

Canada:

https://www.lawdepot.ca/contracts/power-of-attorney-form

United States:

https://www.rocketlawyer.com

These forms are free and accepted in the legal and medical professions. I've included samples of these documents on the following pages.

28 TEMPLATES

Below are some templates you can use to write your own documents related to Medical Directives & Power of Attorney.

ADVANCE MEDICAL DIRECTIVE

This is the Living Will and Medical Directive of

_____,

currently   resident   at

_____.

1. Effective:

a. I recognize that a time may come when by reason of illness or mental incapacity I cannot participate in my medical care or health decisions. This directive will be in effect only while I am unable to make or communicate my own decisions by speaking, by writing, or by gesturing.

2. My Agent:

a. I appoint as my Agent to make personal and health and medical care decisions on my behalf when I no longer have the capacity to make such decisions
_____, currently resident at _____.

b. If _____,
is unwilling or unable to act as my Agent, then I appoint
the first person on the following list who is able and willing to serve as my Alternate
Agent:

_____ of _____
_____ of _____
_____ of _____

c. If my spouse has been designated as an Agent or Alternate Agent above, and if after the execution of this document, my spouse and I are legally separated or divorced, any rights and powers granted to my spouse by this document shall immediately terminate on such legal separation or divorce.

d. Any reference to Agent in this document shall include the meaning Alternate Agent where such Alternate Agent is acting as provided in this document.

3. Power of Agent:

a. I grant to my Agent the full power and authority to make all decisions affecting my health care and living arrangements and I request that my Agent follow my Wishes as indicated in this document. If I have not included instructions on any particular matter that may arise, I hereby empower my Agent to act as he or she thinks best, but in accordance with his or her comprehension of my wishes, values, and beliefs.

b. I grant to my Agent the full power and authority to:
•   sign documents, including but not restricted to releases, permissions, or waivers;
•   review and disclose medical records;
•   hire or discharge caregivers;
•   authorize admission to or release from medical facilities;
•   consent, refuse, or withdraw consent to any form of health care.

4. Visiting Rights:
I hereby request that all medical or care facilities in

which I may be placed give to my Agent primary visiting rights as well as the right to admit or exclude other visitors.

5. My Wishes:

a. If the situation should arise in which there is no reasonable expectation of my recovery from physical or mental disability, then I request that medication be mercifully administered to me to alleviate suffering and that I be allowed to die and not be kept alive by artificial means. I do not fear death itself as much as the indignities of deterioration, dependence, and hopeless pain. In particular, I have the following instructions:

_____

_____

_____

b. If it becomes necessary for a Guardian of my person to be appointed under the appropriate law of the province, then I nominate my Agent, as appointed under clause 2 of this document, as my choice for Guardian.

c. f any dispute arises about the interpretation of my Wishes or about the validity of this Directive, then I encourage my Agent to seek to avoid litigation and to pursue all reasonable ways to resolve the dispute, including mediation.

6. Additional matters:

a. I hereby revoke any previous living wills, personal directives, or advance medical directives.

b. I hereby indemnify and hold harmless my Agent and anyone who acts in good faith at the behest of my Agent in
fulfilling my Wishes as expressed in this document.

7. Signature:

I, _____, of _____, being of sound mind,

confirm that I understand the content of this document

and the power that it gives to my Agent and further confirm that this document represents my Wishes.

DATED at _____,
on this _____ day of
_____, _(year)_____.
SIGNED _____(_____)
in the presence of:

WITNESS _____ (_____)

WITNESS _____ (_____)

ENDURING POWER OF ATTORNEY
I, _____ of the _____
(City, Municipality, Town, District)
of _____ , in the Province/Territory of
_____, state:

    1.   I REVOKE all former Enduring Powers of Attorney previously given by me.

    2.   I   APPOINT (name)_____of the (City, Municipality, Town, District)_____ of
_____ in the Province/Territory of

_____ to be my attorney.

BUT IF my said attorney should refuse to act, or predecease me, THEN I APPOINT _____ of the (City, Municipality, Town, District) _____of _____ in the Province/Territory of _____to be my attorney.

3.   This   power   of   attorney   will   be
EFFECTIVE UPON _____,
   subject   to   the   written   declaration   of
_____.

4.   My attorney has the POWER TO carry
out the following:

29 FINALE

I hope you enjoyed the stories and got something from my book to help you during your caregiving days. If you want to read more about my life go to myloonylife.com. I blog about the things that happen every week because it never ends, not for me.

As I concluded my book and ready to take on my new and exciting life my husband is once again having major heart issues and I guess I'm back full-time caregiving.

This time I'm following my own advice and will seek help when required and make time for me. I maintain a positive outlook on life and look forward to pursuing a career in writing.

ABOUT THE AUTHOR

Alexandra has written a newsletter for her husband's (and her) computer company, every month, for 25 years. Before becoming a full-time caregiver, she was an accountant at a major trucking company and had 30 additional accounting clients. She continues writing on her blog, myloonylife.com and is in the process of writing the first sci-fi book in a trilogy for teens.

Made in the USA
Columbia, SC
18 March 2020